CHEMICAL SENSITIVITY

Consumer Health Library®
Series Editor: Stephen Barrett, M.D.
Technical Editor: Manfred Kroger, Ph.D.

Other titles in this series:

STEPHEN BARRETT, M.D.

CHEMICAL SENSITIVITY
THE TRUTH ABOUT ENVIRONMENTAL ILLNESS

RONALD E. GOTS, M.D., PH.D.

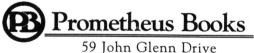
Prometheus Books
59 John Glenn Drive
Amherst, New York 14228-2197

Published 1998 by Prometheus Books

02 01 00 99 98   5 4 3 2

Library of Congress Cataloging-in-Publication Data

Barrett, Stephen, 1933–
    Chemical sensitivity : the truth about environmental illness / Stephen J. Barrett, Ronald E. Gots.
        p.   cm.
    Includes bibliographical references and index.
    ISBN 1–57392–195–5 (cloth : alk. paper)
        1. Multiple chemical sensitivity. 2. Environmentally induced diseases. 3. Medical misconceptions. I. Gots, Ronald E. II. Title.
RB152.6.B37   1998
615.9'02—dc21   97–53181
                                                                          CIP

Printed in the United States of America on acid-free paper

Contents

About the Authors

Stephen Barrett, M.D., a retired psychiatrist who resides in Allentown, Pennsylvania, is a nationally renowned author, editor, and consumer advocate. He is emeritus editor of *Nutrition Forum* newsletter and has been a frequent contributor to *Priorities* magazine and *Consumer Reports on Health*. He is a board member of the National Council Against Health Fraud and chairs its Task Force on Victim Redress. He is medical editor of Prometheus Books and a scientific and editorial advisor to the American Council on Science and Health. He is a scientific consultant and fellow of the Committee for the Scientific Investigation of Claims of the Paranormal (CSICOP) and co-chairs its health claims subcommittee. He operates a clearinghouse for information on health frauds and quackery. He has edited or co-authored forty-four books, including *The Health Robbers: A Close Look at Quackery in America; The Vitamin Pushers: How the "Health Food" Industry Is Selling America a Bill of Goods;* the American Medical Association's *Reader's Guide to "Alternative" Health Methods,* and five editions of the college textbook *Consumer Health: A Guide to Intelligent Decisions.* In 1984, he received the FDA Commissioner's Special Citation Award for Public Service in fighting nutrition quackery. In 1986, he was awarded honorary membership in the American Dietetic Association. His Quackwatch Web site offers comprehensive information on quackery, health frauds, health promotion, and intelligent consumer decision-making. He can reached at (610) 437–1795 or through http://www.quackwatch.com.

    Ronald E. Gots, M.D., Ph.D., is a partner in the International Center for Toxicology and Medicine in Rockville, Maryland, a private, independent consulting resource for occupational and environmental medicine, toxicology, and other comprehensive environmental services. During the past twenty years, he has consulted in thousands of situations involving established or perceived toxic exposure from hazardous waste sites, indoor air contamination, releases from manufacturing facilities, explosions, fires, and other settings. His work helps companies make their products safer for both employees and the environment. He is an adjunct associate professor of toxicology at the Georgetown University School of Medicine and is a member of the Society of Toxicology, the American Public Health Association, the American Industrial Hygiene Association, and the International Society for Regulatory Pharmacology. He has chaired two international conferences on multiple chemical sensitivity. In 1996, he participated in a panel convened by the World Health Organization, the German Federation for the Environment, and the German Health Ministry to develop a consensus on this topic. His writings include six books, several book chapters, and sixty papers in the scientific and forensic literature. His best known book is *Toxic Risks: Science, Regulation, and Perception.* He can be reached at (301) 230–2999.

Acknowledgments

The authors wish to thank the following individuals for their help during preparation of the manuscript:

Project manager	Kathy Deyell
Technical editor	Manfred Kroger, Ph.D.
Associate editor	Jack Raso, M.S., R.D.
Scientific consultants	Robert S. Baratz, M.D., D.D.S., Ph.D.
	Judith Nevyas Barrett, M.D.
	William T. Jarvis, Ph.D.
	Thomas L. Kurt, M.D., M.P.H.
	Herman Staudenmayer, Ph.D.
	Abba I. Terr, M.D.
Legal consultants	Michael Botts, Esq.
	William Custer, Esq.
	Timothy E. Kapshandy, J.D.
	Bonnie Semilof, Esq.
Public policy consultant	Cindy Lynn Richard
Source materials	Paul Benedetti
	Albert Donnay, M.H.S.
Photograph, page 28	Rob Kendrick/AURORA
Drawing, page 29	Pat Linse

1

Be Wary of
Fad Diagnoses

Many Americans believe that exposure to common foods and chemicals makes them ill. This book is about people who hold such beliefs but are *wrong*. Their misbeliefs can be very costly—to health and/or pocketbook—not only for them, but for employers, insurance companies, and others who pay indirectly. Ironically, these accusations are being made at a time when our food supply is the world's safest and our antipollution program is the best we have ever had.

Historical Roots

Throughout history, many people have reported multiple symptoms for which no physical cause was apparent. The ancient Egyptians attributed this problem to displacement or wandering of the uterus. Hippocrates named it *hysteria* (the Greek word for uterus). Nineteenth-century physicians concluded that hysteria's cause was psychological rather than physical. Since that time, patients with physical and mental symptoms and no discernible cause have been given many different labels. During the late nineteenth century, "neurasthenia" was in vogue. Then came vasomotor neurosis, vasoregulatory asthenia, soldier's heart, and Da Costa's syndrome.

Elaine Showalter, Ph.D., a professor of humanities and English at Princeton University, theorizes that symptoms experienced by such

1

patients are culturally determined. In *Hystories: Hysterical Epidemics and Modern Media*, she states:

> Hysterical epidemics require at least three ingredients: physician enthusiasts, unhappy vulnerable patients, and supportive cultural environments. A doctor or other authority figure must first define, name, and publicize the disorder and then attract patients into its community. . . . The most influential doctors of hysteria are also theorists who offer a unified field theory of a vague syndrome, providing a clear and coherent explanation for its many confusing symptoms.[1]

Today's Fads

As medical science deepened its understanding of how the body works, it became clearer that patients fitting the above description were suffering from bodily reactions to stress. However, unconventional physicians began relating such symptoms to glandular disorders and alleged environmental hazards. The glandular conditions include adrenal insufficiency, hypoglycemia (low blood sugar), and hypothyroidism (insufficient thyroid hormone). The environmentally related conditions include candidiasis hypersensitivity; cavitational osteopathosis, chronic fatigue syndrome; food allergies and sensitivities; Gulf War syndrome; Lyme disease; mercury-amalgam toxicity; multiple chemical sensitivity; parasites; and sick building syndrome.[2]

Some of these are recognized diseases that some practitioners diagnose too often. The rest lack scientific recognition. (The table on the opposite page summarizes which is which.) Some practitioners apply one or more of these labels to almost every patient they see.

This book spotlights the "environmental" conditions for which diet and/or chemical exposure are falsely blamed.

• *Multiple chemical sensitivity (MCS)* is a term used to describe people with numerous troubling symptoms they attribute to foods, airborne chemicals, and a long list of other alleged "stressors." Many such people are seeking special accommodations, applying for disability benefits, and filing lawsuits claiming that exposure to common foods and chemicals has made them ill. Their efforts are supported by a small cadre of physicians who use questionable diagnostic and treatment

Perspective on "Fad" Diagnoses

Diagnosis	Scientific Perspective
Adrenal insufficiency	Genuine but rare
Candidiasis hypersensitivity	Not scientifically recognized
Cavitational osteopathosis	Does not exist (see Glossary)
Chronic fatigue syndrome	Common but overdiagnosed
Food allergies and sensitivities	Common but overdiagnosed
Gulf War syndrome	Cause or causes unknown
Hypoglycemia (low blood sugar)	Genuine but overdiagnosed
Hypothyroidism (insufficient thyroid hormone)	Genuine but overdiagnosed
Lyme disease	Genuine but overdiagnosed
Mercury-amalgam toxicity	Not scientifically recognized
Multiple chemical sensitivity	Not scientifically recognized
Parasites	Genuine but overdiagnosed
Sick building syndrome	Not scientifically recognized

methods. Chapters 2 through 4 describe the medical, legal, and political controversies surrounding this dubious diagnosis. Appendices A through F provide scientific and legal reports related to these matters.

• *Candidiasis hypersensitivity* is a diagnosis based on the far-fetched notion that multiple common symptoms result from allergies to the common yeast *Candida albicans*. Its promoters claim that more than eighty million Americans suffer from such a problem. Chapter 5 describes the origin of this diagnosis and why it is invalid. Appendix B includes the leading professional allergy organization's position paper on this subject.

• *Sick building syndrome* is a term used to describe nonspecific symptoms—for which no single cause can be identified—that arise where indoor air quality is under suspicion. Chapter 6 places this term in perspective. Chapter 7 examines claims by people who say that chemical exposure in schools pose a serious problem for children and that food additives cause hyperactivity. These claims are made by MCS promoters and by advocates of the Feingold diet, which is also covered in Chapter 7.

• *Mercury-amalgam toxicity* is said to be a problem for everyone with "silver" tooth fillings. Promoters of this concept claim that significant amounts of mercury escape from the amalgam and poison the body and can cause multiple sclerosis and a long list of other health problems. Chapter 8 debunks such claims. Appendix G shows why the leading anti-amalgamist had his dental license revoked.

• *Gulf War syndrome* is a controversial though ill-defined condition said to involve thousands of Gulf War veterans. Chapter 9 deals with its alleged relationship to MCS.

Many recipients of these diagnoses wind up being financially exploited as well as mistreated. In addition, insurance companies, employers, educational facilities, homeowners, other taxpayers, and ultimately all citizens are being burdened by dubious claims for disability and damages.

Please read on.

References

1. Showalter E. Hystories: Hysterical Epidemics and Modern Media. New York: Columbia University Press, 1997.
2. Barrett S, Herbert V. The Vitamin Pushers: How the "Health Food" Industry Is Selling Americans a Bill of Goods. Amherst, N.Y.: Prometheus Books, 1994.

2

Multiple Chemical Sensitivity: What Is It?

The expression "multiple chemical sensitivity" (MCS) is used to describe people with numerous troubling symptoms attributed to environmental factors. Its underlying concepts were developed by allergist Theron G. Randolph, M.D. (1906–1995), who asserted that patients had become ill from exposures to substances at doses far below the levels normally considered safe. In the 1940s, he declared that allergies cause fatigue, irritability, behavior problems, depression, confusion, and nervous tension in children.[1,2] During this period, he practiced full-time in Chicago and became a staff member of the Northwestern University Medical School and two affiliated hospitals. The foreword to his book *An Alternative Approach to Allergies* indicates that he was charged with being "a pernicious influence on medical students" and subsequently lost his medical school position and hospital privileges.[3]

In the 1950s, Randolph suggested that human failure to adapt to modern-day synthetic chemicals had resulted in a new form of sensitivity to these substances.[4] His concern with foods then expanded to encompass a wide range of environmental chemicals. Over the ensuing years, the condition he postulated has been called allergic toxemia, cerebral allergy, chemical sensitivity, chemical hypersensitivity syndrome, ecologic illness, environmental illness (EI), environmental irritant syndrome, environmental maladaption syndrome, environmentally induced illness, immune system dysregulation, multiple chemical sensitivity, multiple chemical sensitivity syndrome, total allergy

5

syndrome, total environmental allergy, total immune disorder syndrome, toxic encephalopathy, toxic response syndrome, 20th Century disease, universal allergy, and other names that suggest a variety of causative factors. These labels are also intertwined with Gulf War syndrome, sick building syndrome, toxic carpet syndrome, and other politically controversial diagnoses. This multiplicity of names reflects the inability of Randolph's disciples to meaningfully define the condition they postulate.

The complaints associated with these labels include depression, irritability, mood swings, inability to concentrate or think clearly, poor memory, fatigue, drowsiness, diarrhea, constipation, dizziness, mental exhaustion (also called "brain fog" or "brain fag"), lightheadedness, sneezing, runny or stuffy nose, wheezing, itching eyes and nose, skin rashes, headaches, chest pain, muscle and joint pain, urinary frequency, pounding heart, muscle incoordination, swelling of various parts of the body, upset stomach, tingling of the fingers and toes, and psychotic experiences associated with schizophrenia. Proponents claim that virtually any part of the body can have elusive symptoms for which no physical cause can be found. William J. Rea, M.D., who says he has treated more than 20,000 environmentally ill patients, states that they "may manifest any symptom in the textbook of medicine."[5] Another like-minded colleague has said that "MCS patients may well be the human 'canaries' on an increasingly poisoned planet."[6]

Many MCS proponents assert that (1) although one substance may not have an effect, low doses of different substances can add to or multiply one another's effects; (2) hypersensitivity develops when the "total body load" of physical and psychologic stresses exceeds what a person can tolerate; (3) once the process of chemical sensitivity begins, new sensitivities can develop rapidly and from increasingly small exposures; (4) patients often crave and become addicted to foods that make them ill; (5) changes in the degree of exposure can affect the degree of sensitivity to offending substances; (6) hypersensitivities may be related to "immune system dysregulation" or "immunotoxicity" that can be difficult to diagnose and treat; and (7) exposure to environmental pollution often makes people generally susceptible to disease. Some proponents inform patients that they have "an AIDS-like illness." None of these speculations is consistent with scientific knowledge of human physiology, allergy and immunology, pathology, toxicology, or clinical medicine.

Most physicians who diagnose and treat MCS identify themselves as "clinical ecologists" or "specialists in environmental medicine." Clinical ecology is not a recognized medical specialty, is not advocated by standard medical textbooks, and is not a component of medical school or specialty training programs. Environmental medicine is a component of the specialty of preventive medicine (public health), but the theories and practices of clinical ecology are not. To avoid confusion, we refer to advocates of these theories and practices as "clinical ecologists," even though some of them don't describe themselves this way.

Critics of clinical ecology charge that (1) MCS has never been clearly defined, (2) no scientifically plausible mechanism has been proposed for it, (3) no diagnostic tests have been substantiated, and (4) not a single case has been scientifically validated.[7] For these reasons, MCS is not listed as a diagnosis in standard medical textbooks or the *International Classification of Diseases, Ninth Edition, Clinical Modification (ICD-9-CM)*, which is the standard manual used for classifying medical conditions.

Is MCS Definable?

Logic dictates that meaningful research on a condition cannot be conducted until criteria for diagnosing it can be clearly defined. Several definitions of MCS and its synonyms have been proposed, but none has met this standard. For example, the American Academy of Environmental Medicine states:

> Ecologic illness is a polysymptomatic, multi-system chronic disorder manifested by adverse reactions to environmental excitants as they are modified by individual susceptibility in terms of specific adaptations. The excitants are present in air, water, drugs, and our habitats.

Rea and his associates define "chemical sensitivity" as

> an adverse reaction to ambient doses of toxic chemicals in our air, food, and water at levels which are generally accepted as subtoxic. Manifestation of adverse reactions depend on: (1) the tissue or organ involved, (2) the chemical and pharmacological nature of the toxin, (3) the individual susceptibility of the exposed person (genetic make-up, nutritional state, and total load at the time of exposure), (4) the length of the time of exposure, (5) amount and variety of other body stressors (total

load) and synergism at the time of reaction, and (6) the derangement of metabolism that may occur from the initial insults.[8]

In 1985, the ad hoc Committee on Environmental Hypersensitivity Disorders of the Ontario Ministry of Health consulted proponents and reviewed their literature with the hope of defining "environmental hypersensitivity." Although skeptical of clinical ecology's tenets, the committee developed this "working definition":

> Environmental hypersensitivity is a chronic (i.e., continuing for more than three months) multisystem disorder, usually involving symptoms of the central nervous system. Affected persons are frequently intolerant to some foods and they react adversely to some chemicals and to environmental agents, singly or in combination, at levels generally tolerated by the majority. Affected persons have varying degrees of morbidity, from mild discomfort to total disability. Upon physical examination the patient is normally free from any abnormal, objective findings. Although abnormalities of complement and lymphocytes have been reported, no single laboratory test . . . is consistently altered. Improvement is associated with avoidance of suspected agents and symptoms recur with re-exposure.[9]

The label "multiple chemical sensitivity" was coined by Mark Cullen, M.D., professor of occupational medicine at Yale University, who does not identify himself as a clinical ecologist. In a 1987 report, he suggested seven diagnostic criteria: (1) the onset of the problem can be related to one or more documentable environmental exposures, insults, or illnesses; (2) symptoms involve more than one organ system; (3) symptoms recur and abate in response to predictable stimuli; (4) symptoms are elicited by exposures to chemicals of diverse structural classes and toxicologic modes of action; (5) symptoms are elicited by exposures that are demonstrable; (6) exposures that elicit symptoms must be very low (far below average levels known to produce adverse human responses); and (7) no single widely available test of organ-system function can explain the symptoms.[10]

According to a paper published by MCS Referral and Resources (an advocacy organization) and distributed by the National Institute of Environmental Health Sciences (NIEHS):

> Multiple Chemical Sensitivity is a chronic condition marked by greatly increased sensitivity to multiple different chemicals and other irritants. In addition to odor intolerance, some patients also

report increased sensitivity to bright light, sounds, and temperature extremes. MCS may be caused by short-term or chronic exposure to one or more chemicals or other irritants. It can start at any age and includes many often disabling symptoms affecting multiple organ systems, especially the neurological, immune, respiratory, and musculoskeletal systems. . . . The frequency and/or severity of . . . symptoms are made worse by subsequent exposures at even very low doses to a wider range of chemicals and other irritants from a great variety of sources (air pollutants, food additives, fuels, building materials, scented products).[11]

An NIEHS flyer states that MCS involves chemical intolerance, the symptoms of which "appear to be associated with hazardous waste sites, and other community exposures, indoor air pollution, industrial activities, etc."[12]

All of the above definitions differ greatly from those of medically recognized diseases such as diabetes, rheumatoid arthritis, and coronary heart disease, each of which is associated with a clear-cut history, physical findings, and laboratory tests. With MCS, however, the range of symptoms is virtually endless; the onset can be abrupt or gradual and may or may not be linked to any specific exposure or causative factor; and symptoms can vary in intensity, can come and go, and typically do not correlate with objective physical findings and laboratory results.

In short, MCS is little more than a label given to people who do not feel well for a variety of reasons and who share the common belief that chemical sensitivities are to blame. It should not be classified as a disease. It has no consistent characteristics, no uniform cause, and no objective or measurable features. It exists because patients believe it does and doctors validate those beliefs. MCS should really be referred to as a phenomenon rather than a disease.[13]

In 1996, experts who attended an international workshop recommended abandoning the term "multiple chemical sensitivity" because it makes an unsupported judgment on causation. Instead, they suggested "idiopathic environmental intolerances" (IEI), which would have three defining characteristics: (1) an acquired disorder with multiple recurrent symptoms that is (2) associated with diverse environmental factors tolerated by the majority of people and (3) not explained by any known medical or psychiatric/psychologic disorder.[14] In 1997, the board of directors of the American Academy of Allergy, Asthma and Immunology adopted this term in a position statement.[15]

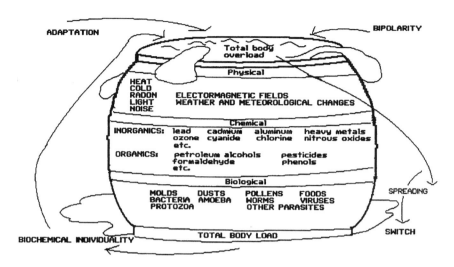

Diagram of clinical ecology theory. Rea's books use dozens of overflowing barrels to depict "pollutant overload."

Elastic Theories

MCS proponents suggest that the immune system is like a barrel that continually fills with chemicals until it overflows and symptoms appear. Some also say that a single serious episode of infection, stress, or chemical exposure can trigger "immune system dysregulation." Potential stressors include practically everything that modern humans encounter, such as urban air, diesel exhaust, tobacco smoke, fresh paint or tar, organic solvents and pesticides, certain plastics, newsprint, perfumes and colognes, medications, gas used for cooking and heating, building materials, permanent press and synthetic fabrics, household cleaning products, rubbing alcohol, felt-tip pens, cedar closets, tap water, and even electromagnetic forces. Rea uses pictures of overflowing barrels to illustrate his concept of "pollution overload."[16]

Randolph's original idea that the symptoms of MCS patients represented a new type of allergy is refuted by the fact that exposure to suspected foods and chemicals usually produces no measurable immunologic response. Although clinical ecologists still tell patients they are "allergic," their theoretical framework has expanded to include immune deficiency, impaired "detoxification," inflammatory responses to free radicals, nasal irritation,[17] "limbic kindling"[18] (see Glossary), neurogenic inflammation,"[19] and several other mechanisms. However, there is no significant evidence to support any of these ideas.

Rea's book *Chemical Sensitivity: Principles and Mechanisms* devotes more than a hundred pages to "nonimmune mechanisms" of MCS.[5] In a preliminary twenty-four-page discussion, Rea delineates six theoretical concepts, none of which is scientifically sound:

• *Total body load*: The sum of all pollutants in the body at one time. These can be biological (pollens, dusts, molds, foods, parasites, viruses, bacteria), chemical (organic or inorganic), psychological (death of a loved one, loss of a job), or physical (heat, cold, electromagnetic radiation, light, radon, positive and negative ions, noise, weather changes). The exposure can be "sudden and massive," such as an accident, toxic exposure, or infection; or it can involve a gradual build-up through low-level exposure to common pollutants.

• *Adaptation*: A mechanism that allows an individual to get used to individual toxic exposures in order to survive them. The body accommodates by adjusting to a new set point with increased output of enzyme-detoxification systems and immune-system enhancement within the physiologic range. Pollutant load may increase in all organs or just one. Over time, adaptation to toxic exposure can result in a long-term decrease in efficient functioning that can shorten life. Because the initial toxic effects may be unrecognizable (masked), repeated exposures may continue that gradually increase total body load and depletion of nutrient fuels

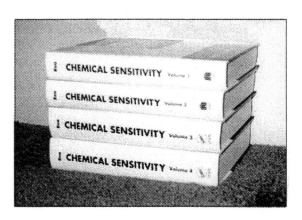

Dr. William Rea's four-volume textbook weighs 13.4 pounds and occupies nearly 3,000 pages.

as the body tries to counteract this build-up. Finally, depressed function occurs, followed by failure of a target organ. Challenge tests performed in an adaptive state are frequently negative. "Deadaptation" can be accomplished by avoiding a suspected substance or reducing total body load for three or four days before testing. But too long a period of avoidance can enable the body to repair its damage and cause a challenge test to be negative.

• *Spreading*: Overload becomes so taxing that a minute toxic exposure to any substance may be sufficient to trigger a response, or autonomous triggering may occur. Thus initial damage by a single chemical can make the body vulnerable to a myriad of unrelated chemicals. Spreading may be due to "failure of the detoxification mechanisms—oxidation, reduction, degradation, and conjugation—brought about by pollution overload," or to "depletion of the nutrient fuels of the enzyme, coenzyme, nutrient fuels, such as zinc, magnesium, all B vitamins, amino acid, or fatty acid." Some chemically sensitive patients may have one organ involved in the disease process for years, only to have dysfunction spread to other organs as their resistance mechanisms break down.

• *Bipolarity*: A "stimulatory/withdrawal reaction" in which a stimulus produces enzyme detoxification, immune changes, and "biological amplification of mediator substances." As a result, a patient may appear "high," as though under the influence of alcohol, or may show no symptoms but still have measurable changes in enzyme and immune induction. Rea states that "observations under environmentally controlled conditions have suggested that this stimulatory/withdrawal reaction leads to the addictive phenomenon which can spill over into cross-reactivity and the spreading phenomenon." With continued exposure to a harmful substance, toxic load increases. After "minutes, months, or years" of overuse, the body's defenses break down, leading to organ failure. Rea also claims that in response to chemical overload, the immune system of sensitive individuals can be stimulated or depressed, or can alternate between the two (a biphasic response).[5]

• *Biochemical individuality*: Individual responses to pollutant exposure are unique and depend on "the differing quantities of carbohydrates, fats, proteins, enzymes, vitamins, minerals, and immune and enzyme detoxification parameters with which an individual is equipped to handle pollutant insults." Thus, when a group is exposed to the a pollutant, one person might develop arthritis, while others develop sinusitis, diarrhea, a bladder infection, asthma, or no disease at all. Biochemical individuality depends on genetic factors, the state of a fetus's nutritional health and "toxic body burden" prior to birth, and the person's nutritional status at the time of exposure. Therefore a patient's reactions to specific foods or chemicals can vary from moment to moment or place to place.

• *Switch phenomenon*: Pollution-stimulated responses change from one organ response to another. This usually occurs acutely, but it may occur over a much longer period. Thus a toxic insult that produces symptoms involving one organ can be the underlying cause of symptoms involving another organ much later, and virtually any sequence of disease could be attributed to MCS.

These concepts, some of which originated with Theron Randolph, purportedly explain why (1) some individuals are sensitive to doses below known toxic thresholds, (2) symptoms may not be related to known toxicities of specific chemicals, (3) established mechanisms of action may not apply, (4) symptoms may show up long after a chemical exposure, (5) the duration of symptoms may not be related to the amount of chemical exposure, and (6) negative challenge tests are not accurate. In short, Rea postulates that exposure to just about anything—in any dosage or concentration—can cause just about any health problem, at any time, and that challenge testing may not consistently detect the problem.

In *The Healthy School Handbook*, Rea warns that children are more vulnerable than adults. He states:

Over 2,000 metabolic genetic defects have now been identified, in addition to long-known anatomic ones. It is reasonable to assume that most children have one or more of these defects, which are time bombs, waiting for the right environmental triggers to manifest their pathology.[20]

Regarding pregnancy, he further states:

> The activity of the mother . . . may result in a bioconcentration of the toxics in the fetal tissue (i.e., if the mother drinks her coffee from a styrofoam cup, she may retain one part per billion of the styrofoam while her fetus may retain two or three parts per billion). Such a bioconcentration can occur for many chemicals, thus increasing the fetus's toxic load and causing more vulnerability to any new environmental exposure. . . . Excess toxic load depletes nutrients such as vitamins, minerals, and amino acids, thus allowing vulnerability to disease, learning disability, and poor brain function.[20]

Rea's theories may seem plausible to laypersons, but experts are not impressed. Some of the processes he describes cannot be measured, and some are not testable because they involve too many variables. Although he uses scientific-sounding terms, his theories clash with current medical knowledge. There is no known mechanism whereby low levels of chemicals or chemicals of widely varied structure can interact adversely with numerous organ systems.[21] There is no plausible mechanism that can link widely disparate responses in different individuals to the same chemicals or whereby sensitivity to one chemical can confer sensitivity to hundreds of others. Moreover, if the "total body load" concept were valid, the "sum" of small amounts of many unrelated chemicals (as well as infections and psychological stresses) would have the same effects as massive doses of single chemicals—which is not true. Chemicals, including those used as drugs, have specific effects that depend on the amounts to which individuals are exposed.[22] When chemicals have different basic structures, their toxic effects usually differ too. If individual responses were unique and unpredictable, it would be impossible to develop useful drugs.[13]

A Typical Example

Several years ago, shortly after beginning work at a newly constructed day-care center, three women reported brief episodes during which they smelled the odor of sewer gas. Each reported smelling the gas for several seconds, a few times a day, but not every day. One said that the odor sometimes made her vomit and that she also developed diarrhea, burning of her face, and muscle soreness, which were diagnosed as a viral infection. A few weeks later, all three women developed additional symptoms and were diagnosed as having a sinus infection. Although the odors stopped soon afterward and testing detected no unusual levels of airborne chemicals in the center, they continued to feel sick whenever they worked there.

A septic tank hookup may have been responsible for brief migration of sewer gases into the building. However, there is no reason to believe that this made these women ill. Similar odors are part of our everyday experience—when we move our bowels. Nevertheless, the women concluded that the odors had harmed them. They began experiencing palpitations, dizzinesss, lightheadedness, and various other symptoms even when not at work. They sought additional medical help and were examined at a major university medical center, where the occupational medicine physicians evaluating them declared that they had MCS. One recommended psychiatric care. The other told them that there was no available treatment for their condition. Certain that they had been poisoned and that there was little hope, the women then sought the care of a clinical ecologist who recommended sauna treatments, dietary modification, and avoidance of all chemical exposures. The women became progressively unable to function, joined an MCS support group, and consulted an attorney.

A year later, when examined by an occupational medicine specialist and a psychiatrist, the women remained dysfunctional despite "treatment" that had cost thousands of dollars. The diagnosis was clear. The women were suffering from panic attacks related to worrying about their health and aggravated by being told they had MCS.

The above pattern is typical of MCS patients. Perception of a hazard leads to fear of chemical exposure. Coincidental symptoms become associated with the perceived hazard. An MCS diagnosis leads to generalized avoidance of chemicals and withdrawal from customary activities. The symptoms continue despite this advice.

The Scientific View

The key issue in the multiple chemical sensitivity controversy is whether MCS is primarily psychogenic or chemically-induced. That is, are symptoms caused by an emotional response to perceived chemical exposures or by actual physical injury resulting from an interaction between chemical agents and organ systems?

The question is often asked whether this determination is necessary. Two arguments are typically advanced against it. First, the ultimate cause of symptoms is irrelevant; rather a sufferer requires compassion and should not be a pawn in causality debates. Second, clear distinctions between psychogenic and chemically induced disorders are not readily made. While both of these arguments have some merit, neither eliminates the need to classify patients properly. It is true that sufferers need to be treated compassionately; but how they are treated and who treats them should be determined by the underlying cause of the symptoms. A psychogenic origin would warrant behavioral therapy. A chemically induced cause would warrant avoidance and exposure-control methodologies.

Many experts have studied MCS patients and concluded that their basic problem is psychologic rather than physical.[23] The best current data suggest that certain psychologic factors predispose individuals to develop symptoms and to seek out someone who will provide a "physical" explanation of their symptoms.[24,25] Many of these patients suffer from somatization disorder, an emotional problem characterized by persistent symptoms that cannot be fully explained by any known medical condition, yet are severe enough to require medical treatment or cause alterations in lifestyle.[26] Some are paranoids who are prone to believe that their problems have outside causes.[27] Others suffer from depression, panic disorder,[28] agoraphobia, hyperventilation syndrome,[29] or other anxiety states that induce bodily reactions to stress.[30]

The term "multiple chemical sensitivity" does these patients a disservice by suggesting that their symptoms are caused by chemicals when they are not. Chapter 3 looks closely at this problem.

References

1. Randolph TG. Fatigue and weakness of allergic origin (allergic toxemia) to be differentiated from 'nervous fatigue' or neurasthenia. Annals of Allergy 3:418–430, 1945.
2. Randolph TG. Allergy as a causative factor in fatigue, irritability and behavior problems in children. Journal of Pediatrics 31:560–572, 1947.
3. Moss RW. Foreword to Randolph TG, Moss RW. An Alternative Approach to Allergies. New York: Bantam Books, 1982.
4. Randolph TG. The specific adaptation syndrome. Journal of Laboratory and Clinical Medicine 48:934, 1956.

5. Rea W. Chemical Sensitivity: Tools of Diagnosis and Methods of Treatment. Boca Raton, Fla.: CRC Press, 1996.
6. Ziem G. Multiple chemical sensitivity: My clinical experience and response to the Bascom Report. In Chemical Hypersensitivity Syndrome Study: Comments of the Review Committee. Baltimore: Maryland Department of the Environment, 1989.
7. Staudenmayer H, Selner JC. Failure to assess psychopathology in patients presenting with chemical sensitivities. Journal of Occupational Medicine 37:704–709, 1995.
8. Rea WR and others. Considerations for the diagnosis of chemical sensitivity. In Talmage DW and others. Biologic Markers in Immunotoxicology. Washington, D.C.: National Academy Press, 1992.
9. Thomson GM and others. Report on the ad hoc Committee on Environmental Hypersensitivity Disorders. Toronto: Ontario Ministry of Health, 1985.
10. Cullen MR. The worker with multiple chemical hypersensitivities: An overview. State of the Art Review. Occupational Medicine 2:655-661, 1987.
11. Donnay, A. Recognition of multiple chemical sensitivity. MCS Referral and Resources, Baltimore, Nov. 1994.
12. National Institute of Environmental Health Sciences. Multiple chemical sensitivity. Undated flyer distributed in 1997.
13. Gots RE. Multiple Chemical Sensitivities: What Is It? North Bethesda, Md.: Risk Communication International, Inc., March 31, 1993.
14. Conclusions and recommendations of the workshop on multiple chemical sensitivities (MCS), February 21–23, 1996. Regulatory Toxicology and Pharmacology 24:S188–S189, 1996.
15. Terr AI, Bardana EJ, Altman LC. Position statement: Idiopathic environmental intolerances (IEI). American Journal of Allergy and Immunology (in press).
16. Rea WJ: Chemical Sensitivity: Principles and Mechanisms. Boca Raton, Fla.: Lewis Publishers, 1992.
17. Meggs WJ and others. Nasal pathology and ultrastructure with chronic airway inflammation (RADS and RUDS) following an irritant exposure. Clinical Toxicology 34:383–396, 1996.
18. Bell IR, Miller CS, Schwartz GE. An olfactory-limbic model of MCS syndrome: possible relationships to kindling and affective spectrum disorders. Biological Psychiatry 32:218–242, 1992.
19. Meggs WJ. Neurogenic inflammation and sensitivity to environmental chemicals. Environmental Health Perspectives 101:234–238, 1993
20. Rea WJ. Why children are more susceptible to environmental hazards. In Miller NL, editor. The Healthy School Handbook: Conquering the Sick Building Syndrome and Other Environmental Hazards in and around Your School. Washington, D.C.: National Education Association, 1995:39–49.
21. Gots RE. Multiple chemical sensitivities: Distinguishing between psychogenic and toxicodynamic. Regulatory Toxicology and Pharmacology 24:S8–S15, 1996.

22. Pirages SW, Richard CL. Multiple chemical sensitivities. AIHA Journal 58:94–97, 1997.
23. Kurt TL. Multiple chemical sensitivities: A syndrome of pseudotoxicity manifest as exposure perceived symptoms. Clinical Toxicology 33:101–105, 1995.
24. Simon GE, Katon WJ, Sparks PJ. Allergic to life: Psychological factors in environmental illness. American Journal of Psychiatry 147:901–906, 1990.
25. Gots RE. Hypothesis and practice: Autointoxication and MCS. Regulatory Toxicology and Pharmacology 18:2–12, 1993.
26. American Psychiatric Association. Diagnostic and Statistical Manual, 4th Edition. Washington, D.C.: American Psychiatric Association, 1994.
27. Rosenberg SJ, Freedman MR, Schmaling KB, and others. Personality styles of patients asserting environmental illness. Journal of Occupational Medicine 32:678–681, 1990.
28. Binkley KE, Kutcher S. Panic response to sodium lactate infusion in patients with multiple chemical sensitivity syndrome. Journal of Allergy and Clinical Immunology 99:570–574, 1997.
29. Leznoff A. Provocative challenges in patients with multiple chemical sensitivity. Journal of Allergy and Clinical Immunology 99:438–442, 1997.
30. Bock KW, Birbaumer N. MCS (multiple chemical sensitivity): Cooperation between toxicology and psychology may facilitate solutions of the problems: commentary. Human & Experimental Toxicology 16:481–484, 1997.

3

MCS: Dubious Diagnosis
and Treatment

The fact that MCS has not been meaningfully defined does not deter clinical ecologists from diagnosing it—typically in all or nearly all of their patients. Their diagnostic evaluation usually includes an "ecological oriented history," a physical examination, and laboratory tests. However, the diagnosis may be based entirely on what the patient reports. In addition to standard items, the history-taking procedure may include a nonstandard questionnaire that emphasizes dietary habits and exposure to environmental chemicals.

The nature and purpose of the physical examination are unclear. Dr. William Rea's textbook, for example, does not specify how the examination should be done. The book states that hives, eczema, bleeding into the skin, bruises, edema (swelling of the skin), and coldness of hands and feet, are "extremely common signs," and that "holes in the fingernails, ridges and white spots on the nails, and hangnails are often present." Rea also says that MCS patients often exhibit bad breath, belching, mouth ulcers, abdominal tenderness, tenderness over the bladder, back tenderness, vaginal discharge, prostate tenderness, acne, and many other physical findings and illnesses.[1] The book claims that "pallor of the skin, which ranges from pale to deep yellow," is a definite sign of chemical sensitivity and appears in most MCS patients. Besides that, he lists no physical sign or combination of signs that is specific to MCS. Actually, there is no reason to believe that chemical sensitivity is a likely cause of skin pallor any of the other symptoms that Rea mentions.

Do you have environment-related illness?
Take the following questionnaire and find out.

1. Does exposure to cigarette smoke and/or perfume cause you to experience symptoms?
2. Do you notice more symptoms at work than at home—or visa versa?
3. Do you have frequent headaches or migraines?
4. Has your productivity level decreased substantially over the past few months or years?
5. Do you have allergy symptoms and/or repeated bouts of sinusitis, bronchitis, nasal polyps, chronic ear and throat infections, or ringing in the ears?
6. Have you been diagnosed with chronic fatigue syndrome, Epstein Barr Virus, cytomegalovirus, herpes virus—or do you have an overwhelming fatigue?
7. Does your work or do your hobbies expose you to toxic minerals, metals, or chemicals?
8. Have you been diagnosed with irritable bowel syndrome or do you have frequent nausea, bloating, constipation, or diarrhea?
9. Do you experience chronic muscle and joint aches and pains—or have you been diagnosed with fibromyalgia?
10. Do you routinely have your home and/or yard sprayed with pesticides?
11. Do you frequently experience forgetfulness, difficulty concentrating, or numbness and tingling?
12. Have you had a positive ANA (antinuclear antibody) test or do you have M.S., lupus, rheumatoid arthritis, an autoimmune disease, or a history of cancer?
13. Do you have or have you had breast implants, and did you see a correlation between implantation and the beginning of your symptoms?
14. Has any type of metal been used in implants or joint replacements in your body? Can the onset of your health problems be traced to the time of the implant?
15. Do you have named cardiovascular disease without knowing the cause?
16. Miscellaneous questions or concerns: _____

If you answered "yes" to three or more of these questions, you could have environment-related illness. By recording your answers and sending this form on to EHC-D—we'll give you feedback on your responses.

The Environmental Health Center–Dallas Web site invites visitors to answer this questionnaire by e-mail. What percentage of American adults do you think would answer yes to at least three questions? What percentage with three or more yesses do you think need treatment for "environmental sensitivity?"

Some standard laboratory tests may be performed, mainly to rule out other causes of disease. Standard allergy test results are often normal.

The test clinical ecologists consider most important is called provocation-neutralization. During this procedure, the patient is asked to report any symptoms that develop after various concentrations of suspected substances are administered under the tongue (sublingually) or injected into the skin (intradermally). If symptoms occur, the test is considered positive and various concentrations are given until a dose is found that "neutralizes" the symptoms. Various other chemicals, hormones, food extracts, and other natural substances may be prescribed as "neutralizing" agents.

"Neutralization" superficially resembles the desensitization process used by allergists. However, allergists test and treat with substances that produce measurable, objective, allergic responses, whereas clinical ecologists base their judgments on subjective responses (what the patient reports).

Clinical ecologists differ about how provocation and neutralization should be done.[2] The observation period is generally said to be ten minutes, but reported times have ranged from seven to ninety minutes. Whereas some practitioners increase the amount of the test substance in the "neutralizing" dose, others lower it. Rather than devise and test standard protocols, clinical ecologists have generally relied on personal experience, testimonials, and anecdotal evidence. Moreover, they accept test results without establishing whether they are consistent or reproducible.

After reviewing the test records of MCS patients, toxicologist William J. Waddell, M.D., reported that the following responses were considered evidence of sensitivity: "yawn, burp, sniffle, raw throat, face pressure, muscle tremor, itch, droopy eye muscle, burning feeling, eye twitch, woozy head, eye itch, sleepy, less sleepy, cough, nervous, headache, lousy feeling, heart pounding, feel bad, neck noise, groggy, restless legs, and weak." He noted that the responses could differ from one test to another with the same chemical and had no objective significance:

> The salient problem with MCS is that there is no consistent and specific effect from exposure to any specific chemical. This does not allow for any objective test for any disease entity which might be caused by the chemicals as indicated by the theory of

MCS. The effects of exposure to chemicals as defined today by MCS are subjective, and no report is available to convincingly demonstrate that these effects would not have occurred merely by chance.[3]

Waddell also concluded: (1) the MCS hypothesis (exposure to any chemical may or may not produce any illness after exposure to the same or any other chemical) was not specific enough to be testable, (2) the hypothesis contradicts fundamental principles of toxicology, (3) current testing procedures for MCS are so subjective that they are useless, (4) there is no evidence that the responses attributed to MCS differ from those that would occur merely by chance, and (5) the MCS literature attaches an emotional bias to chemicals.

Many clinical ecologists use tests related to immune function or exposure to specific chemicals. Samples of blood, urine, fat, and hair may be examined for various environmental chemicals, the most common of which are organic solvents, hydrocarbons, pesticides, insecticides, and heavy metals. Other blood tests may assess immunoglobulins, other immune complexes, lymphocyte counts, and "antipollutant enzyme" levels.[4] Some of these tests lack an accepted protocol and have not been standardized, and none has been demonstrated to have a consistent pattern of alteration in MCS patients.[5]

Elimination and rotation diets may be used with the hope of identifying problematic foods. An elimination diet may begin with a one-week "washout" or fast during which only spring water is consumed. Single-food challenges may also be used. In severe cases, Rea's patients may spend several weeks in an environmental unit intended to remove them from exposure to airborne pollutants and synthetic substances. After fasting for several days, these patients are given "organically grown" foods and gradually exposed to environmental substances to see which ones cause symptoms to recur. The other services offered at Rea's clinic include nutritional counseling, fitness testing, biofeedback, stress management, osteopathic manipulation, cranial manipulation, oxygen therapy, nutrient therapy, homeopathy, acupuncture, and eye-lens manipulation. His facility also offers treatment for children with "allergies/ sensitivities, attention deficit hyperactivity disorder, learning disorders, chronic ear infections, asthma, behavior problems, and other chronic problems of childhood including arthritis, cardiomyopathy (a disorder of the heart muscle), and vascular dysfunction."[6]

Some MCS-related programs are based on blood tests that can detect chemicals in concentrations of parts per billion. This enables levels too low to be clinically significant to be misinterpreted as evidence of unusual and harmful chemical exposure.[7] If any "toxin" level is interpreted as abnormal, the patient will be advised that "detoxification" or "purification" can wash the undesirable chemicals from the body. The regimens may include exercise, sauna treatments, showers, massage, herbal wraps, megavitamin therapy (usually including several grams of niacin per day), self-administered "desensitization" injections, and the use of water and air purifiers.[8,9] An astute reporter has pointed out that people can't sweat out toxins because the sweat glands are not connected to the liver or any other organ that process toxins.[10] Moreover, high doses of niacin tend to interfere with detoxification by the liver.

Some clinical ecologists claim that PET or SPECT scans can detect brain abnormalities caused by exposure to environmental substances. The Society of Nuclear Medicine Brain Imaging Council disagrees.[11]

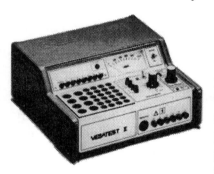

A few practitioners who consider themselves clinical ecologists use a fancy galvanometer to diagnose "energy imbalances" or "allergies" and select homeopathic remedies or other products to correct the alleged problems. These devices merely measure the electrical resistance of the skin, which reflects how moist it is and how hard the operator presses a probe against the patient's skin. Skin moistness is easily influenced by emotions, but the most important factor is how hard the probe is pressed. The test results have nothing whatsoever to do with allergies, chemical sensitivities, the state of the patient's health, or any type of energy imbalance. Although the FDA considers such devices "a significant risk" to the public, it has done little to curb their use.

Provocation-Neutralization Debunked

Two scientific studies have demonstrated that provocation testing and neutralization treatment are not valid. Both found that patients reacted similarly to the test substances and placebo.

In 1971, two researchers reported on tests performed by five experienced clinical ecologists. Each of the patients had tested positive during provocation testing with special preservative-free extracts of food or alcohol, the contents of which were known to the clinical ecologist. During the experiment, the clinical ecologist was handed either the extract or a dilute saltwater solution (saline), the contents of which were known only to another physician who observed but did not participate in the procedure. Based on the patient's reactions, the clinical ecologists were then asked to judge whether the administered material was the extract or the placebo. The extracts were correctly identified in twenty-four of thirty-four trials (70.6 percent). However, the salt-water solution relieved the patient's symptoms in twenty-eight of forty trials (70 percent), indicating that symptom relief was not related to any allergy-causing substance in the extracts.[12]

In the early 1980s, researchers at the University of California (UC) observed similar test results in a study funded by the Society for Clinical Ecology and the American Academy of Otolaryngic Allergy (another proponent group). The tests took place in the offices of seven clinical ecologists who had been treating the patients. During three-hour sessions, the patients received three injections of suspected food extracts and nine of normal saline. Sixteen patients were tested once, and two were tested twice. In ordinary tests, these patients had consistently reported symptoms when exposed to food extracts and no symptoms when given saline injections. Under double-blind conditions, however, when neither they nor their doctors knew what was in the injections, they developed symptoms with sixteen (27 percent) of the food-extract injections and forty-four (24 percent) of the saltwater injections. The symptoms elicited by both types of injections were identical and included itching of the nose, watery or burning eyes, plugged ears, a feeling of fullness in the ears, ringing ears, dry mouth, scratchy throat, an odd taste in the mouth, tiredness, headache, nausea, dizziness, abdominal discomfort, tingling of the face or scalp, tightness or pressure in the head, disorientation, difficulty breathing, depression, chills, coughing, nervousness, intestinal gas or rumbling, and aching legs. The results clearly demonstrated that the patients' symptoms were placebo reactions. The study also tested the claim that "neutralizing" doses of offending allergens can relieve the patient's symptoms. All seven patients who were "treated" during the experiment had equivalent responses to extracts and saline. The researchers noted:

It is regrettable that every patient undergoing challenge or provocative testing is not tested in a double-blind fashion so that the effect of suggestion or anxiety on the end points could be evaluated. If they were so tested, the problems with the validity of the method that we found would have been discovered decades ago.[13]

Don L. Jewett, M.D., who led the UC study, provided additional perspective at a 1992 conference on MCS:

Some may find it unusual that an orthopedic surgeon has had clinical and investigative experience with the hypersensitivity syndrome. My experience occurred in three ways: as a patient, as a treating physician, and as a scientific investigator. As a patient, I have had lifelong allergies, which became worse during an especially difficult period of my life. Traditional allergy shots produced some mild, but unsustained, improvement. I then started treatment under a clinical ecologist and ultimately spent five weeks in a Dallas environmental control unit. I ended with a diagnosis of "universal reactor," 70 different injection substances, and a change (but not a decrease) in symptoms. . . .

After this I began seeing patients in a "sensitivity clinic" that I ran within the Orthopedic Clinic at the University of California, San Francisco. I treated patients with diet changes (four-day rotation diet). Some patients seemed to experience significant positive effects. Such results encouraged me to formulate a long-range plan to definitively prove the hypothesis that small amounts of substances to which we are commonly exposed can result in symptoms (at least in some patients at some times). Because the expected positive result was likely to have a significant impact on medical practice, I devised a scientifically rigorous study that both proponents and opponents agreed was a fair and appropriate double-blind test of symptom provocation by injections. However, the study showed provocation testing to be totally unreliable as a method for determining sensitivity, and so I began to doubt the validity of this diagnostic and therapeutic approach. . . .

My role as an investigator is limited to the above-cited study because proponents immediately dropped association with me when the negative results were presented to a national meeting of the Society for Clinical Ecology.

Jewett later observed that patients who described their most troubling problems as interpersonal often did well with counseling, but most who considered their problem physical did poorly because they found it "difficult or impossible to stop their compulsive search for a medical or technological solution to their problem."[14]

Environmental Chamber Tests

Allergist John C. Selner, M.D., and psychologist Herman Staudenmayer, Ph.D., of Denver, Colorado, have treated hundreds of "MCS" patients during the past seventeen years. They are not clinical ecologists and reject clinical ecology theories and practices. They believe that although some people are very sensitive to various microorganisms, noxious chemicals, and common foods, there is no scientific evidence that an immunologic basis exists for *generalized* allergy to environmental substances. Using well-designed double-blind tests, they have demonstrated that people said to be "universal reactors" may develop multiple symptoms in response to test procedures without being allergic to any of the individual substances administered. One of their reports describes how they used an environmental chamber to evaluate twenty patients who had multiple symptoms attributed to hypersensitivity to workplace and domestic chemicals. These patients believed that they were reactive or hypersensitive to low-level exposure to many chemicals. Some had previously been evaluated and managed by clinical ecologists and diagnosed with MCS. During nonblinded tests, these patients consistently reported symptoms they had associated with exposure at work, at home, or elsewhere.

The environmental chamber enabled the patients to encounter measured amounts of purified air, compressed gasses, and air containing specific chemical concentrations, without knowing which situation was which. During the controlled test periods, patients were randomly exposed to (1) chemicals to which they believed they were sensitive; (2) the same chemicals with their odors masked by another odor such as peppermint spirit, anise oil, cinnamon oil, or lemon oil; (3) just the odor used for masking; or (4) clean air. A total of fifty-seven active and eighty-eight sham challenges were performed. After each test period the patients were asked whether they thought they had been exposed to a suspected chemical or to clean air. The patients were monitored for objective signs (such as skin reactions) and were also asked to report symptoms experienced during the test and up to three days later. None of the twenty patients demonstrated a response pattern implicating the chemicals supposedly responsible for their symptoms. Eighteen reported no symptoms at least once when the suspect chemical was present. Fifteen reported symptoms at least once when the suspect chemical was absent.[15] In other words, many MCS patients react to their feelings about the test, rather than to the substance in question.[16]

Questionable Products

The treatments clinical ecologists recommend are as questionable as their diagnoses. One observer has commented that the variety of what they prescribe "seems limited only by their imagination and resourcefulness."[17] The usual approach emphasizes avoidance of suspected substances and involves lifestyle changes that can range from minor to extensive. Generally, patients are instructed to modify their diet and to avoid such substances as scented shampoos, aftershave products, deodorants, cigarette smoke, automobile exhaust fumes, and clothing, furniture, and carpets that contain synthetic fibers. Extreme restrictions can involve wearing a charcoal-filter mask, using a portable oxygen device, staying at home for months, or avoiding physical contact with family members. Many patients are advised to take vitamins, minerals, and other dietary supplements. Neutralization therapy, based on the results of provocative tests, can involve administration of chemical extracts under the tongue or by injection.

Shirley W. Kaplan, M.A., who says she has suffered for more than ten years, has described her vulnerability this way:

> If an individual is chemically sensitive, his or her whole world is up for grabs. Everything the . . . patient eats, breathes, or otherwise comes in contact with has to be evaluated as a possible source of symptoms. For me, finding alternative foods and

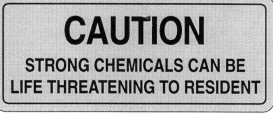

CAUTION
STRONG CHEMICALS CAN BE
LIFE THREATENING TO RESIDENT

Sign for use at the residence of an MCS patient.

nontoxic manufactured products was a minor difficulty compared to contemplating major modifications in my home. Most difficult was the way in which the illness became a significant challenge to be reckoned with in every relationship and activity. Suddenly not only my own but everyone else's perfume, detergent, home and office became a potential problem for me.[18]

MCS patients typically portray themselves as immunologic cripples in a hostile world of dangerous foods and chemicals and an uncaring medical community. In many cases, their life becomes centered around their illness. Various companies cater to their concerns by offering such items as "organic" foods; odor-free personal products; special clothing, household products, and building materials; and even specially outfitted travel trailers. A recent article in *Reason* described how one woman wore a protective mask while shopping and another woman hung her mail on a clothesline for weeks before reading it, to allow the "toxins" in the ink to dissipate.[10]

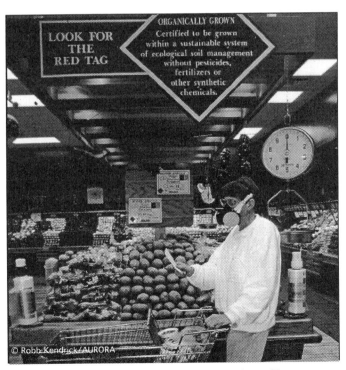

Some MCS patients wear a mask to filter
the air they breathe when away from home.

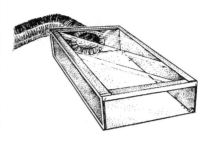

Desktop reading box. Made of tempered safety glass and aluminum, its purpose is to shield the user from chemicals in ink or paper. The item to be read is placed inside the box. The tube contains an exhaust fan that is vented through an outside window. The 1995 American Environmental Health Foundation catalog offered the box for $295 plus $35 for a glass side, $35 for a hinged glass door, and additional expense for shipping.

In 1975, Rea founded the American Environmental Health Foundation in Dallas, Texas. Its 1995 catalog stated that the foundation had "funded over 30 major medical research projects and provided environmentally safe products to patients and to the public-at-large." The catalog offers air filters, bedding, educational materials, paints, building materials, children's supplies, clothing, ecological masks, electromagnetic shielding, "full spectrum" lighting, furniture, oxygen masks, personal air purifiers, pet supplies, pollution detection kits, reading boxes (outfitted with an exhaust fan to suck away gasses presumably emitted from a newspaper, typewriter, or laptop computer), saunas, water filtration systems, water test kits, and more than 150 dietary supplement products. The supplements are said to be hypoallergenic and made by manufacturers who use "the purest products and methods . . . and, wherever possible, use organically grown plants for their sources." The products include *Mood Elevator, Powder Carrots, Powder Potato*, and two brands of shark cartilage.

An ad in the American Academy of Environmental Medicine's 1996–1997 membership directory offers homeopathic products for "stress, both physical and emotional," "cellular repair," and "organ systems clearing and specific biotoxin eradication i.e., chemicals, metals, viruses." The manufacturer, HVS Laboratories of Naples, Florida, states that "every one of your patients is affected by these cell damaging toxins." The products are said to be prepared "electromagnetically," to "add to the electromagnetic vitality of the body," and to "complement all other modalities." HVS recommends "clearing" the patient at least annually, but states that some practitioners prescribe weekly "preventive" doses "in an effort to minimize toxic buildup."[19] Despite the apparently booming marketplace, homeopathic products have no proven value for any health problem (see Glossary).

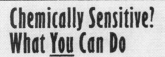
Ads for various MCS-related products and services.

Critical Scientific Reports

Many prominent professional organizations and scientific panels have concluded that clinical ecology and its associated concepts are—at best—speculative and unproven.

• The California Medical Association Scientific Board Task Force on Clinical Ecology conducted an extensive literature review and held a hearing at which proponents testified. Its report states (1) no convincing evidence supports the hypotheses on which clinical ecology is based; (2) clinical ecologists have not identified specific, recognizable diseases caused by low-level environmental stressors; and (3) the methods used to diagnose and treat such undefined conditions have not been proven effective. The task force concluded that "clinical ecology does not constitute a valid medical discipline" and should be considered "experimental" only when its practitioners adhere to scientifically sound research protocols and inform their patients accordingly. The task force also expressed concern that unproven diagnostic tests can lead to misdiagnosis, which results in patients being denied other supportive treatment, becoming psychologically dependent, and believing they are seriously and chronically impaired.[20]

• The ad hoc Committee on Environmental Hypersensitivity Disorders established by the Minister of Health of Ontario, Canada, received submissions, heard testimony from many professionals and laypersons, observed practitioners at work, and issued a 500-page report describing the concepts of clinical ecology and the evidence, if any, supporting them.[21] An expert panel then reviewed this report and concluded that "scientific support for the mechanisms that have been proposed to underlay the wide variety of dysfunctions are at best hypothetical. Moreover, the majority of techniques for evaluating the patients and the treatments espoused are unproven."[22] The table on the next page summarizes data from patient reports to the committee.[23]

• In 1986, the American Academy of Allergy, Asthma and Immunology (AAAAI), which is the nation's largest professional organization of allergists, published a position statement based on an extensive literature review and comments by its members. The statement said:

> The idea that the environment is responsible for a multitude of human health problems is most appealing. However, to present such ideas as facts, conclusions or even likely mechanisms without adequate support is poor medical practice. . . .

There are no immunologic data to support the dogma of the clinical ecologists.... The suggestion that neutralization therapy can provide rapid relief within minutes or hours cannot be supported by controlled clinical studies or immunologic data....

Advocates of this dogma should provide adequate studies ... which meet the usually accepted standards for scientific investigation.[24]

In 1997, the AAAAI reviewed the evidence again and concluded that "a causal connection between environmental chemicals, foods, and/or drugs and the patient's symptoms is speculative and not based on the results of published scientific studies."[25]

• The American College of Physicians (ACP) has issued a position paper concluding that "there is no body of evidence that clinical ecology treatment measures are effective."[2] An accompanying editorial in the same journal notes that its promotion has many characteristics of a cult and that its treatment approach should not be considered harmless.[26]

• The Canadian Psychiatric Association's position statement on environmental hypersensitivity acknowledges that patients diagnosed as

Experiences of "Environmental Hypersensitivity" Patients

Average number of years ill (51 reports)	11
Total types of symptoms	161
Total treatment measures	62
Total types of diagnostic tests	34
Substances said to be allergenic	143
Had allergies as a child	59
Average number of medical practitioners seen	6
Total types of practitioners seen	38
Average yearly cost (18 reports)	$4,463
Financial burden reported	73

Except as noted, the data were compiled from a random sample of 147 of 614 individual submissions received from patients, family members, or friends. Source: Committee on Environmental Hypersensitivity Disorders.[42]

environmentally sensitive experience subjective discomfort and sometimes disability. The Association concluded, however, that "there is not sufficient evidence to state that environmental pollutants or food additives cause the complaints subsumed under the term 'environmental hypersensitivity.' "[27]

• The American Medical Association Council on Scientific Affairs has concluded:

> Until . . . accurate, reproducible, and well-controlled studies are available . . . multiple chemical sensitivity should not be considered a recognized clinical syndrome. . . .
>
> Based on reports in the peer-reviewed scientific literature . . . (1) there are no well-controlled studies establishing a clear mechanism or cause for [MCS]; and (2) there are no well-controlled studies providing confirmation of the efficacy of the diagnostic and therapeutic modalities relied on by those who practice clinical ecology.[28]

• The Board of the International Society of Regulatory Toxicology and Pharmacology (ISRTP) has concluded:

> Current scientific information reports no clinical, laboratory, or other objective support for the proposition that MCS represents a clinically definable disease entity. The theories claiming to unify this condition as a toxicologically mediated disorder transgress basic principles of toxicology and clinical sciences. These violations include the allegations that: (1) a toxic response to one chemical can lead to a "sensitivity" to all other chemicals; (2) "petrochemicals" and "man-made" chemicals somehow differ in their toxicological potentials from "natural" chemicals; (3) a chemical may induce widespread symptoms associated with all organ systems; and (4) the manifestations of toxic responses to chemicals may vary widely and completely from individual to individual. Because these claims are both unproven and inconsistent with the current state of scientific knowledge, the ISRTP adopts the position that "MCS and its disorders, known as ecological illness and environmental illness, cannot be considered an organically based toxicological disease process."[29]

A National Research Council (NRC) subcommittee has concluded that hypersensitivity has an immunologic basis, but "multiple chemical sensitivity (MCS) syndrome" does not.[30] (In other words, although some people are sensitive to small doses of one or a few specific chemicals, the idea that people become generally hypersensitive to chemicals has no scientific foundation.) The subcommittee also noted that the controversy surrounding the diagnosis of MCS cannot be resolved until MCS is clearly and measurably defined and then explored with well-designed studies. After a workshop at which proponents discussed possible research protocols, the NRC warned again that meaningful research on "multiple chemical sensitivity" cannot be conducted until clear criteria for such a diagnosis can be defined.[31] Despite this, MCS proponents tout NRC's involvement as evidence that their beliefs and practices are legitimate.

A passage in the NRC's 1992 report unfairly criticized allergist Abba I. Terr, M.D., who had authored the American College of Physicians position paper on clinical ecology. Two MCS proponents used this passage to attempt to pressure the college to withdraw its 1989 position statement.[32] The ACP refused and protested to NRC, which issued an erratum with the criticism of Terr deleted.[33]

In 1996, an NRC committee concluded that there is no convincing evidence that electromagnetic fields (EMFs) have any adverse effects on health. Among other things, the report noted no evidence to show that EMFs can alter the function of cells at levels of exposure common in residential settings.[34]

Case Studies

Many patients are relieved when a clinical ecologist offers what they think they need and encourages them to participate actively in their care. However, the treatment they receive may do them far more harm than good.

• Carroll M. Brodsky, M.D., Ph.D., professor of psychiatry at the University of California (San Francisco) School of Medicine, described the recruitment process in a report on eight people who, following diagnosis by a clinical ecologist, had filed claims for injury primarily by airborne substances. He concluded that they were "adherents of physicians who believed that symptoms attributed by orthodox physicians to psychiatric causes are in fact due to common substances in air, food, and water." He also stated that clinical ecologists

> neither promise nor give hope of eliminating the offending condition, and the patients do not seem to expect it. . . . [They] seem content with their condition and with the reassurance that

their symptoms have a physical cause. . . . Yet we must also recognize that these patients have had symptoms for many years, and whether seen as neurasthenic, hypochondriacal, or phobic, they are among the most resistant and difficult to treat. . . . These patients search for healers who will provide them with an explanation of their experiences and symptoms that makes sense to them and fulfills a number of psychological needs.[35]

The fact that some clinical ecologists believe that they themselves have MCS has been described as "a powerful bonding tool which snares patients into a . . . cult interdependence in which facts are irrelevant."[36]

• In 1986, Abba I. Terr, M.D., an allergist affiliated with Stanford University Medical Center, reported on fifty patients who had been treated by clinical ecologists for an average of two years. Most of these patients had made a workers' compensation claim for industrial illness. Although all had been diagnosed as "environmentally ill," Dr. Terr could find no unifying pattern of symptoms, physical findings, or laboratory abnormalities. Eight of the patients had not developed symptoms until after they had consulted a clinical ecologist because they had been worried about exposure to a chemical. Eleven had had symptoms caused by preexisting problems unrelated to environmental factors, and thirty-one had multiple symptoms. Their treatments included dietary changes (74 percent of the patients), food or chemical extracts (62 percent), an antifungal drug (24 percent), and oxygen given with a portable apparatus (14 percent). Fourteen of the patients had been advised to relocate to a rural area, and a few were given vitamin and mineral supplements, gamma globulin, interferon, female hormones, and/or oral urine. Despite treatment, twenty-six patients reported no lessening of symptoms, twenty-two felt worse, and only two had improved.[37]

In 1989, Terr reported similar observations on ninety patients, including forty who had been covered in the previous report.[38] Although one or more of over fifty sources of chemicals at their workplace had been blamed for the patient's problem, Terr noted that the testing process did not usually include extracts of the workplace materials that were presumed responsible. He also noted that thirty-two of the ninety patients had been diagnosed as suffering from "candidiasis hypersensitivity," a diagnosis that the American Academy of Allergy, Allergy and Immunology considers "speculative and unproven" (see Chapter 5). Since provocation-neutralization tests had played a major role in the misdiagnosis of most of the patients he examined, Terr pointed out that scientific studies have shown it is unreliable. He believes that although exposure to chemicals can cause disease, it is unlikely that the diagnostic and treatment methods of clinical ecology are effective. He also believes that its methods and theories appear to cause unnecessary fears and lifestyle restrictions.

• Dr. William Rea's Environmental Health Center (EHC) in Dallas, Texas, was founded in 1974 and now has clinics in Chicago; Texarkana, Texas; and Halifax, Nova Scotia. During the 1980s, Canadian investigators who examined the files of 2,000 of Rea's patients reported that only four had tested negative for environmental sensitivity, and those four were found to have cancers. The reviewers concluded that Rea's test procedures lacked appropriate controls and the patients were assumed to have environmental hypersensitivity mainly by being referred to the unit.[39]

• In 1989, a reporter from the syndicated television program "Inside Edition" visited Rea's clinic as a patient. The reporter truthfully told Rea that he had been feeling more tired than usual, that he was having headaches that could be relieved by aspirin, that his eyes had been getting red more often than usual, and that his shoulder still hurt from an accident several months ago. Rea said that all the symptoms could be due to allergies and ordered a lengthy series of skin tests.

Before visiting Rea, the reporter had been checked by Raymond G. Slavin, M.D., past president of the American Academy of Allergy, Asthma and Immunology, who had found no evidence of allergy. After the reporter returned from his visit to Rea, Slavin said that Rea's testing was a waste of money because the reporter's story did not provide a legitimate basis to suspect that his symptoms were due to allergies. Slavin also said that the skin reactions produced by the testing were caused by irritation from the injected chemicals rather than by allergies. "Inside Edition" reported that treatment at Rea's facility cost thousands of dollars and that he referred many of his patients to a trailer court near Dallas where "environmentally safe" cottages and trailers could be rented for $500 per week. Rea also has operated an inpatient unit at a hospital in Dallas. Rea's patient manual—about seventy-five pages long—contains detailed instructions about choosing foods and avoiding environmental chemicals.[40]

• A research team from the state of Washington conducted immunologic and psychologic tests of forty-one MCS patients and thirty-four patients with chronic musculoskeletal problems. The immunologic tests revealed no significant differences between the two groups. The MCS patients tended to have higher levels of psychologic distress and a greater tendency to report "medically unexplained" physical symptoms.[41]

• Philip Witorsch, M.D., and colleagues from the Georgetown University Medical Center evaluated sixty-one MCS cases, examining forty-one of them directly and reviewing the records of the rest. In no case were there any objective physical or laboratory findings that correlated with the subjective complaints. Among the forty-one who were seen, all fit established criteria for at least one psychiatric diagnosis.[42]

• MCS patients commonly report difficulty concentrating, remembering, or thinking clearly. However, researchers at the Robert Wood Johnson Medical School performed standardized neuropsychological tests and found no significant differences in cognitive function among thirty-six MCS patients, eighteen chronic fatigue patients, and eighteen apparently healthy control subjects.[43]

• Donna E. Stewart, M.D., associate professor of psychiatry and of obstetrics and gynecology at the University of Toronto assessed eighteen "20th Century disease" patients referred to the university's psychiatric consultation service and concluded:

> Virtually all had a long history of visits to physicians, and their symptoms were characteristic of several well known psychiatric disorders. . . . It is important that patients with a wide range of diagnosable and treatable psychiatric conditions not receive a misdiagnosis of 20th-century disease and thereby embark on a prolonged, socially isolating, expensive and often harmful course of ecologic treatment that reinforces their invalidism.[44]

• Ronald E. Gots, M.D., Ph.D., has reviewed the medical records of more than a hundred MCS patients and concluded:

> Unlike many "alternative medical practices," the diagnosis of MCS begins a downward spiral of fruitless treatments, culminating in the withdrawal from society and condemning the sufferer to a life of misery and disability. This is a phenomenon in which the diagnosis is far more disabling than the symptoms.[45]

One situation Gots reviewed involved a family of four whose house had undergone routine treatment by an exterminator. At the time the treatment was administered, the mother had respiratory symptoms—most likely caused by an influenza virus—which worsened after the exterminator's visit. Soon afterward, her husband and two children, ages nine and seven, also became infected. Having read about the allegedly widespread health effects of chemicals, the mother began to think that the pest-control treatment had caused her family's symptoms. After recovering from the viral illness, she developed fatigue, headaches, abdominal discomfort, and several other symptoms, which she believed also were caused by pesticide exposure. And she concluded that the others were similarly afflicted. The woman consulted a clinical ecologist who agreed that she and her family had developed MCS as a result of pesticide exposure. At his suggestion, the children took notes to school asking that they not be allowed to work with crayons or paints. The parents also demanded that the children be excused from school on days when the floors or tables were polished, or extermination services were administered. Eventually, the mother's demands for special consideration became insupportable and she withdrew her children from class, choosing instead to instruct them herself at home. The family also moved to a secluded cabin in the woods.

• Psychiatrist Donald W. Black, M.D., and colleagues at the University of Iowa College of Medicine reported that the prevalence of major psychiatric disorders among twenty-six "environmental illness" (EI) patients was more than twice as high as that of a control group. The researchers concluded that patients receiving this diagnosis may have one or more commonly recognized psychiatric disorders that could explain some or all of their symptoms.[46]

These researchers later described how the misdiagnosis involved can produce psychosocial, financial, occupational, and psychological complications. The psychosocial complications usually stem from recommendations to avoid contact with offending agents. As a result, patients become socially constricted or reclusive. The financial cost can be enormous; for example, a patient may be instructed to add a "safe" room to his house, or even to rebuild the entire house. Relocating can be very expensive, particularly if it involves quitting a job or moving long distances to seek a pollutant-free environment. Occupational complications can arise when a person is advised to quit a job or stop working because of presumed exposure on the job. The researchers concluded:

> Perhaps the major disadvantage to receiving a diagnosis of EI is that it deprives the subject of an appropriate medical or psychiatric diagnosis and access to proven therapies. For example, a person with depression could receive appropriate [medication].

. . . Furthermore, the diagnosis of EI can be psychologically damaging because it reinforces illness behavior and promotes the idea that a patient is an immunologic cripple; this erroneous belief is then reinforced and validated by the support network that has developed around EI.[47]

Black has also described the cases of four patients with hypochondriacal beliefs that they were chemically hypersensitive. All had been instructed not to work (or to change their line of work) and to avoid social activities. Black concluded: "In addition to misattributing symptoms to a diagnosis of questionable validity, the clinical ecologists involved with these patients failed to recognize treatable psychiatric disorders."[48]

• A committee sponsored by the government of Nova Scotia examined the medical records of eighty-six patients said to be "environmentally hypersensitive." In every case, the panel was able to make a standard medical or psychological diagnosis. The committee concluded there was no evidence to confirm the existence of "environmental illness."[49]

• By 1985, Drs. Selner and Staudenmayer had tested more than a hundred patients in their environmental unit. In a lengthy report, they concluded (1) people do exist who are very sensitive to various microorganisms, noxious chemicals, and common foods; (2) the key question is whether multisystem disease can be caused by generalized allergy to environmental substances; (3) when a physician is confronted by a patient claiming to be "allergic to everything," the diagnosis can usually be traced to the influence of a proponent of clinical ecology; (4) there is no scientific evidence that an immunologic basis exists for such a symptom pattern; (5) clinical ecologists assume that if even a trace of any chemical is found in the patient's environment, that chemical can be held responsible for any symptom; (6) clinical ecologists appear to lack the motivation or intellectual capacity to test their theories scientifically; (7) clinical ecologists offer a philosophy of certainty, often reassuring patients during an initial phone contact that their diagnosis is obviously ecologic disease; (8) patients with genuine allergies to noxious chemicals do not have multisystem complaints without associated physical or laboratory findings; (9) many patients with symptoms of "environmental illness" find "healers" who tell them they are "universal reactors" to environmental substances; (10) this explanation of their experience and symptoms makes sense to them and enables them to avoid facing their

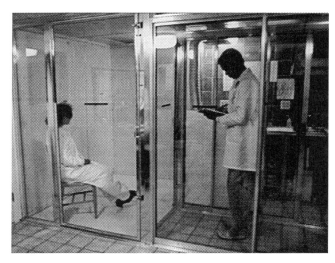

Environmental chamber used by Drs. Selner and Staudenmayer. Using an open challenge, patients were exposed to low levels of chemicals they believed were responsible for their symptoms. If symptoms occurred, retesting was done under double-blind conditions.

real problem—which is psychological; (11) most people said to be "universal reactors" develop multiple symptoms in response to the testing process without being allergic to any of the individual substances administered; and (12) once patients understand that this can happen, psychotherapy may cure them.[43]

One of Selner and Staudenmayer's successful patients was a forty-five-year-old woman who had been troubled by headaches, generalized pain, depression, confusion, and abdominal discomfort. After a four-day standardization period in which her environment was controlled without dietary alteration, she experienced remarkable relief from all of her symptoms except the abdominal discomfort. She was placed in a challenge booth and, under blinded conditions, exposed to a sham challenge of clean air. Her symptoms recurred immediately and lasted several hours. After two days of fasting (with spring water), she had no symptoms. She then was challenged with a tiny amount of Fuller's earth (an inert substance) in four gelatin capsules. She had an immediate reaction that left her with a severe gastrointestinal upset, vertigo (dizziness), severe weakness, and mental confusion that lasted for more than forty-eight hours. A diagnosis of somatization was made, and the situation was explained to her. Accepting this explanation, she entered an outpatient psychotherapy program, lost nearly all of her symptoms, achieved employment success, and resolved many things that had been troubling her emotionally.[43]

Actually, the idea that common symptoms could have an emotional basis has been known to medical scholars for more than a century. One physician who understood this was John Noland MacKenzie, M.D., an ear, nose and throat specialist in Baltimore. In 1886, he wrote about a thrity-two-year-old woman who believed she was sensitive to dozens of environmental factors, particularly the odor of roses. The woman suffered from bouts of depression, malaise, impaired mental ability, general irritability, sneezing, and a long list of other burdensome complaints. MacKenzie did not believe that rose pollen was responsible for the woman's symptoms, so he obtained a realistic-looking artificial rose and carefully cleaned it to be sure that it contained no trace of foreign matter. During the woman's next visit, after determining that she felt unusually well, he took the rose from behind a screen and held it in his hand while they talked. Almost immediately, the woman developed itching of her throat; itching, tearing, and redness of her eyes; a runny nose; hoarseness; and shortness of breath. She even developed swelling of the membranes inside her nose. When the deception was revealed, the woman expressed amazement, but within a few days she became able to smell genuine roses without developing her usual symptoms.

This woman was fortunate because her doctor realized that her symptoms were not solely due to allergy. Once she understood this, she stopped reacting to the sight or odor of roses.[50] A recent court case illustrates what can happen when the patient's true problem goes untreated. In 1991, a jury in New York City awarded $489,000 in actual damages and $411,000 in punitive damages to the estate of a man who committed suicide at age twenty-nine after several years of treatment by a clinical ecologist. Testimony at the trial indicated that the patient was a paranoid schizophrenic who thought "foods were out to get him." This type of mental problem may respond well to antipsychotic medication. However, the testimony indicates that the doctor had diagnosed the man as a "universal reactor" and advised that, to remain alive, he had to live in a "pure" environment, follow a restrictive diet, and take dietary supplements.[51]

Another serious problem is the disruption that occurs when family members disagree about the value of "ecological" treatment. In one case we know about, a teenage girl troubled by fatigue was diagnosed as sensitive to foods, chemicals, and electromagnetic fields by clinical ecologists whose tests, treatments, and recommended household modifications cost $100,000 during a one-year period. Although the girl's condition worsened, she and her mother had complete faith in the treatment and wanted to continue it. The girl's father, who concluded that the treatment was futile, was forced to choose between continuing to pay for it or antagonizing his wife and daughter, whom he deeply loved. With great reluctance, he filed for divorce in order to protect himself against financial ruin.

References

1. Rea W. Chemical Sensitivity: Tools of Diagnosis and Methods of Treatment. Boca Raton, Fla.: CRC Press, 1996.
2. Terr AI and others. Clinical ecology. Annals of Internal Medicine 3:168–178, 1989.
3. Waddell WJ. The science of toxicology and its relevance to MCS. Regulatory Toxicology and Pharmacology 18:13–22, 1993.
4. Rea WR and others. Considerations for the diagnosis of chemical sensitivity. In Talmage DW and others. Biologic Markers in Immunotoxicology. Washington, D.C.: National Academy Press, 1992.
5. Sparks PJ, Daniell W, Black DW and others. Multiple chemical sensitivity syndrome: I. Case definition, theories of pathogenesis, and research needs. Journal of Occupational Medicine 36:718–730, 1994.
6. Environmental Health Center—Dallas Web site (http://www.ehcd.html), Oct. 1997.
7. Sparks PJ, Daniell W, Black DW and others. Multiple chemical sensitivity syndrome: II. Evaluation, diagnostic testing, treatment, and social considerations. Journal of Occupational Medicine 36:731–737, 1994.
8. Kurt TL, Sullivan TJ III. Toxic agoraphobia. Annals of Internal Medicine 112:231, 1990.
9. Kurt TL. Sauna-depuration: Toxicokinetics. Presented at the Second Annual Environmental Medicine Conference, Aspen Colorado, Sept. 8, 1995.
10. Fumento M. Sick of it all. Reason 28(2):20–26, 1996.
11. Society of Nuclear Medicine Brain Imaging Council. Ethical clinical practice of functional brain imaging. Journal of Nuclear Medicine 37:1256–1259, 1996.
12. Kailin EW, Collier R. 'Relieving' therapy for antigen exposure. JAMA 217:78, 1971.
13. Jewett DL, Fein G, Greenberg MH. A double-blind study of symptom provocation to determine food sensitivity. New England Journal of Medicine 323:429-433, 1990.

14. Jewett DL. Diagnosis and treatment of the hypersensitivity syndrome. Toxicology and Industrial Health 8(4):111–117, 1992.
15. Staudenmayer H, Selner JC, Buhr MP. Double-blind provocation chamber challenges in 20 patients presenting with "MCS." Regulatory Toxicology and Pharmacology 18:44–53, 1993.
16. Staudenmayer H. Multiple chemical sensitivities or idiopathic environmental intolerances: Psychophysiologic foundation of knowledge for a psychogenic explanation. Journal of Allergy and Clinical Immunology 99:435–437, 1997.
17. Black DW. Environmental illness and misdiagnosis—a growing problem. Regulatory Toxicology and Pharmacology 18:23–31, 1993.
18. Kaplan SW. It's not all in their heads: Managing the psycho-social aspects of sick school building syndrome. In Miller NL, editor. The Healthy School Handbook: Conquering the Sick Building Syndrome and Other Environmental Hazards in and around Your School. Washington, D.C.: National Education Association, 1995:51–59.
19. Kratz AM. Questions . . . answers. Naples, Fla.: HVS Laboratories, undated flyer distributed Feb. 1997.
20. Wiederholt WC and others. Clinical ecology—a critical appraisal. Western Journal of Medicine 144:239–245, 1986.
21. Thomson GM and others. Report of the ad hoc Committee on Environmental Hypersensitivity Disorders. Toronto: Ontario Ministry of Health, 1985.
22. Zimmerman B and others. Report of the Advisory Panel on Environmental Hypersensitivity. Ontario: Ministry of Health, 1986.
23. Report of the ad hoc Committee on Environmental Hypersensitivity Disorders—Appendices. Toronto: Ontario Ministry of Health, 1985.
24. Anderson JA and others. Position statement on clinical ecology. Journal of Allergy and Clinical Immunology 78:269–270, 1986.
25. American Academy of Allergy, Asthma, and Immunology. Idiopathic environmental intolerances (IEI): Position statement. American Journal of Allergy and Immunology (in press).
26. Kahn E, Letz G. Clinical ecology: environmental medicine or unsubstantiated theory? Annals of Internal Medicine 111:104–106, 1989.
27. Scientific Council of the Canadian Psychiatric Association. CPA Statement on hypersensitivity. Ottawa, March 1990.
28. Estes EH Jr, Coble YD and others: Clinical ecology. JAMA 268:3465–3467, 1992.
29. Board of the International Society of Regulatory Toxicology and Pharmacology. Report of the ISRTP Board. Regulatory Toxicology and Pharmacology 18:79, 1993.
30. Talmage DW and others: Biologic Markers in Immunotoxicology. Washington, D.C.: National Academy Press, 1992.
31. Samet J and others: Multiple Chemical Sensitivities: Addendum to Biologic Markers in Immunotoxicology. Washington, D.C.: National Academy Press, 1992.
32. Davis ES, Lamielle M. Letter to Denman Scott, M.D., April 18, 1992.

33. Talmadge DW. Biologic Markers in Immunotoxicology: Erratum to page 135. Attachment to letter to Abba I. Terr, M.D., Oct. 2, 1992.
34. Stevens CF and others. Possible Health Effects of Exposure to Residential Electric and Magnetic Fields. Washington, D.C.: National Academy Press, 1996.
35. Brodsky CM. 'Allergic to everything': A medical subculture. Psychosomatics 24:731–742, 1983.
36. Selner JC, Staudenmayer H. The relationship of the environment and food to allergic and psychiatric illness. In Young SH and others, editors. Psycho-biological Aspects of Allergic Disorders. New York: Praeger, 1986:102–146.
37. Terr AI. Environmental illness: A clinical review of 50 cases. Archives of Internal Medicine 146:145–149, 1986.
38. Terr AI. Clinical ecology in the workplace. Journal of Occupational Medicine 31:257–261, 1989.
39. McCourtie D. An overview. In Chronic Diseases in Canada: Environmental Sensitivities Workshop, Ottawa, Ontario, May 24, 1990. Ottawa: Health and Welfare Canada, 1991:7–8.
40. Rea WJ. Outpatient Information Manual. Dallas: Environmental Health Center, 1988.
41. Simon GE, Daniell W, Stockbridge H, and others. Immunologic, psychological, and neuropsychological factors in multiple chemical sensitivity. A controlled study. Annals of Internal Medicine 119:97-103, 1993.
42. Witorsch P and others. Multiple chemical sensitivity: Clinical features & causal analysis in 61 cases. Presented at the 1995 North American Congress of Clinical Toxicology Annual Meeting, Rochester, N.Y., Sept. 17, 1995.
43. Fiedler N, Kipen HM, DeLuca J, and others. A controlled comparison of multiple chemical sensitivities and chronic fatigue syndrome. Psychosomatic Medicine 58:38–49, 1996.
44. Stewart DE. Psychiatric assessment of patients with "20th-century disease." ("total allergy syndrome"). Canadian Medical Association Journal 133:1101–1106, 1985.
45. Gots RE. Multiple chemical sensitivities—Public policy. Clinical Toxicology 33:111–113, 1995.
46. Black DW, Rathe A, Goldstein RB. Environmental illness. A controlled study of 26 subjects with '20th century disease.' JAMA 264:3166–3170, 1990.
47. Black DW, Rathe A, Goldstein RB. Measures of distress in 26 "environmentally ill" subjects. Psychosomatics 34:131–138, 1993.
48. Iatrogenic (physician-induced) hypochondriasis: Four patient examples of "chemical sensitivity." Psychosomatics 37:390–393, 1995.
49. Medical Post, Oct. 13, 1992, p. 49.
50. Mackenzie JN. The production of the so-called "rose cold" by means of an artificial rose. American Journal of Medical Science 91:45–57, 1886.
51. Medical malpractice: Treatment of paranoid schizophrenia by "clinical ecology"—wrongful death—punitive damages. New York Jury Verdict Reporter 10(23):1–2, 1991.

4

MCS: Political and Legal Issues

Rejection of MCS concepts by the scientific community has done little to dampen the enthusiasm of clinical ecologists or decrease the loyalty of their patients. Many of them belong to professional or support groups that promote their interests.

Professional Organizations

About four hundred clinical ecologists belong to the American Academy of Environmental Medicine (AAEM).[1] This organization, founded by Theron Randolph, M.D., in 1965 as the Society for Clinical Ecology, is composed mainly of medical and osteopathic physicians. Its conferences, despite their questionable content, have been accepted for continuing education credits by the American Medical Association and the American Academy of Family Physicians. AAEM's journal was published in the 1980s as *Clinical Ecology* and renamed *Environmental Medicine* in 1991. During the late 1980s, the journal announced that the paper on which it was printed had been changed because several readers had complained that the old paper had made them ill. In the same issue, the editor complained that he was not receiving enough acceptable manuscripts to maintain a quarterly schedule. The publication frequency subsequently decreased.

Clinical ecologists also play a significant role in the American Academy of Otolaryngic Allergy (AAOA), which was founded in 1941 by Randolph and others who espoused diagnostic and treatment procedures that mainstream allergists regarded as invalid. AAOA has about 2,300 members, most of whom are board-certified otolaryngologists.[2] The percentage of members who espouse the practices of clinical ecology is unknown, but some AAOA seminars are taught by leading clinical ecologists. AAOA has endorsed the use of provocation and neutralization testing.[3]

The MCS Support Network

Two sociologists who have suggested that MCS is chemically induced have described a common MCS mindset:

> People with MCS . . . believe that at any moment their relative state of illness and wellness is a function, in part, of the activities and practices in others. Important, perhaps critical, to a person's management of MCS is her ability to persuade other people that they are partly responsible for her misery and must change if she is to successfully manage her symptoms. People with MCS must narrate their symptoms in order to survive.[4]

Several organizations offer a ready outlet for such expression.

The Human Ecology Action League (HEAL), founded in 1977, is composed mainly of laypersons and has chapters and support groups in about a hundred cities. It distributes physician and supplier referral lists, maintains a World Wide Web site, and publishes *The Human Ecologist,* a quarterly magazine of news and advice for patients and their families. HEAL's travel guide lists suitable facilities, but advises MCS travelers to check carefully ahead of time and to send their own cleaning supplies in advance so they can be used to prepare the room.[5] HEAL also tells members how to press insurance companies to pay for their medical care, which usually costs thousands of dollars.

Earon S. Davis, J.D., M.P.H., a former executive director of HEAL, published the bimonthly *Ecological Illness Law Report* from 1982 through 1988 and operated a referral service that attracted two hundred interested attorneys. In 1987, at his urging, the Association of Trial Lawyers of America voted to establish a clearinghouse on "ecological illness" and its legal aspects. Davis recently stated that he is no longer involved in MCS-related activities.

The National Center for Environmental Health Strategies (NCEHS), of Voorhees, New Jersey, is a membership organization that was started in 1986. Its now-defunct newsletter, *The Delicate Balance,* was said to have achieved an international distribution exceeding four thousand. Its founder and president, Marie Lamielle, says that she started the group after an exposure to toxic chemicals, when she "found that no public agency or private organization could answer my questions or advocate for me."

The Chemical Injury Information Network (CIIN), of White Sulfur Springs, Montana, was founded in 1990 and has over five thousand members. It publishes *Our Toxic Times*, a monthly newsletter for people "suffering from chemically related health problems." A CIIN brochure lists 150 items in its "MCS symptom checklist," but notes: "Unfortunately this is not a complete list."[6] In 1996 the newsletter announced that MCS advocates had joined forces with environmental activists to form the Chemical Injury Council, whose primary purpose is litigation. Its initial aims include:

> examination of the unethical practices of independent medical examiners, decertification of self-insured employers that consistently injure their workers, multiple plaintiff actions against employers that chemically injure their employees, and multiple plaintiff actions against state agencies that consistently engage in unfair and inconsistent determinations of claimants' cases.[7]

CIIN's research arm, called the Environmental Access Research Network (EARN), publishes *Medical & Legal Briefs,* a bimonthly newsletter edited by Cindy Duerhing. EARN also does computer searches, provides photocopies and telephone consultations, and maintains referral lists of attorneys and expert witnesses.

MCS advocates have also sought sympathy and political support by attacking what they portray as the "big, bad chemical industry." The Chemical Injury Litigation Project, coordinated by MCS activist Julia Kendall, helped MCS patients find physicians and lawyers. According to press reports, she and about two dozen others wore respirators and shouted "perfume stinks" during a demonstration outside the hotel housing the 1994 annual convention of the Cosmetic, Toiletry and Fragrance Association.[8] She is reported to have said, "Basically . . . we want to destroy the [fragrance] industry."[9] She died in July 1997.

MCS Referral & Resources, of Baltimore, Maryland, publishes reports, makes referrals, operates a clearinghouse, and engages in "public advocacy devoted to the diagnosis, treatment, accommodation and prevention of multiple chemical sensitivity disorders." Its executive director is Albert Donnay, MHS, and its president and medical director is Grace Ziem, M.D., Dr.P.H. Its publications include "Who Recognizes Multiple Chemical Sensitivity?" a quarterly report listing "legislative and administrative policies and court decisions that recognize MCS as a legitimate disease and or disability."

The National Institute of Environmental Health Sciences (NIEHS), a component of the National Institutes of Health, has adopted what appears to be a "neutral" policy. Packets distributed by its Environmental Health Clearinghouse contain proponent literature as well as scientific articles. One item written by a NIEHS official even states that MCS is a syndrome of chemical intolerance, the symptoms of which "appear to be associated with hazardous waste sites, and other community exposures, indoor air pollution, industrial activities, etc."[10] NIEHS has supported MCS research, workshops, and other conferences. In fiscal years 1994 through 1996, it provided at least $29 million for research projects classified as MCS-related. However, many of the projects (such as "Inner City Cockroach Allergen Reduction Trial" and "Radiosensitive Target in the Early Mouse Embryo") appear irrelevant.

Reasonable Accommodation?

In 1991, federal regulators ruled that MCS can be considered a disability under the Americans with Disabilities Act (ADA). The act defines disability as a "physical or mental impairment that substantially limits one or more of the major life activities" of an individual.[11] Its intended purpose was to prevent discrimination against qualified employees based on their disability. To be qualified, an individual must be able to do the job with or without reasonable accommodations. The law does not specify MCS as a disability and does not require employers to provide speculative ineffective accommodations.[12] Claims are decided case by case.

Citing the ADA, NCEHS has lobbied to persuade employers and government agencies to adopt policies that "accommodate employees and members of the public disabled by chemical barriers." Its lengthy list of recommendations includes: (1) better ventilation systems; (2) no use of air fresheners; (3) no indoor use of pesticides except in emergencies;

(4) no use of synthetic lawn chemicals near the workplace; (5) no smoking in or near the workplace; (6) purchase of the "least toxic/allergenic" building materials, office furnishings, equipment, and supplies; and (7) employee prenotification for "construction and remodeling activities and toxic cleaning activities such as the use of paints, adhesives, and solvents, carpet shampoos and floor waxes." Many MCS patients have demanded that their workplace be totally free of odors. MCS sufferers have also argued for prohibition of perfumes, colognes, and fragrant hygiene products in the workplace. However, there has been no ruling about whether such prohibition would be a reasonable accommodation.

In 1994, the University of Minnesota School of Social Work posted a notice that anyone wearing a scented product would be asked to leave. Administrative officials said the policy was voluntary. The action was taken in response from claims that two people had MCS. The school's general counsel said that even if it could be determined that they were disabled, the policy could not go beyond reasonable accommodation.[13]

HEAL advises that children with MCS may have rights under both the ADA and the Individuals with Disabilities Act of 1975. Its newsletter has provided detailed strategies for seeking accommodations. In one example, it recommended seating the child next to an open window, steam-cleaning new carpeting, installing a portable air cleaner, and damp-mopping floors instead of waxing them. In another example, it advised parents to demand home-bound instruction unless the school is willing to designate an empty classroom as a "safe room" for use by a single MCS child.[14]

In 1992, the U.S. Department of Housing and Urban Development (HUD) concluded that multiple chemical sensitivity and environmental illness are handicaps within the meaning of the Federal Fair Housing Amendments Act. HUD memoranda have stated that individuals so handicapped are entitled to "reasonable accommodations" to be determined case by case.

Attempts to accommodate chemically sensitive people are often futile. The most publicized example is that of Ecology House, an eight-unit "safe house" constructed in San Rafael, California. HUD contributed $1.2 million toward the project's $1.8 million total cost. The tenants were selected by lottery from about one hundred applicants around the country. To qualify, they had to have medical certification that they were disabled from MCS and had to earn less than $20,450 per year.[15] Although the building was intended to be free of synthetic chemicals, most of the initial tenants said it still made them sick.[16]

In 1996, as part of an investigation by ABC's "20/20," a healthy ABC employee and her healthy sister-in-law visited Dr. Grace Ziem. After a brief physical exam and some questions, they completed a sixteen-page questionnaire and were told they were chemically sensitive. Each was charged $900 and advised to get $3,000 worth of lab tests. One was also advised to move out of New York City and the other was warned not to get pregnant. The program reported that, after moving into a Virginia townhouse complex, one of Ziem's patients filed a series of complaints and lawsuits charging that her community had discriminated against her by failing to accommodate her chemical sensitivity. HUD told the community board that since the woman was chemically disabled, her special needs must be accommodated. The program stated that the woman had complained about the pesticides and fertilizers used by her neighbors, paint on mailboxes, cars idling near her home, and leaf blowers, and that the neighbors' legal defense costs had exceeded $150,000. Legal action of this type enables a single individual to infringe on the rights of many others.

The idea of protecting "sensitive" persons can be appealing when presented as protecting everyone from unwanted exposures.[17] However, it is unfair for regulatory agencies, legislative bodies, and the courts to attempt to prevent or to compensate for idiosyncratic reactions and experiences.

MCS in Court

Many people who believe that chemical exposure has harmed their health have taken legal action consistent with this belief. One case involved clinical ecology's founder, Theron Randolph, M.D., and his wife, Janet. In 1977, a federal tax court ruled that their extra expense for "organically grown" foods was tax-deductible as a medical expense. The Randolphs claimed that Janet experienced mental confusion, crossed eyes, and difficulty in walking when she inhaled or ingested contaminants, and that Theron had suffered from loginess (sluggishness), malaise, headaches, nausea, and anorexia due to contaminated foods.

One area of great concern to MCS proponents is whether insurance companies will pay for their treatment, which can be quite expensive. Advice on how to press for such payment is available from MCS advocacy groups. Many patients seeking reimbursement wind up filing a lawsuit. Such suits can be expensive to defend and may trigger an award for punitive damages if a jury concludes that an insurance company has acted in "bad faith" in refusing to pay for clinical ecology treatment.

Claims and lawsuits are also being filed to collect workers' compensation and Social Security Disability. Although awards are limited and individual claims may not be expensive to defend, some cases involve many workers who claim they were made ill by low-dose exposure to chemicals in the workplace. Some courts have recognized MCS as a compensable occupational disease or a disability. Even when the court does not recognize MCS as a disease, it may award benefits to a plaintiff considered disabled by a somatization disorder or other psychological condition.[18] Many MCS advocates disapprove of basing benefits on such psychological diagnoses. In a recent court case, the Social Security Administration recognized MCS as a medically determinable impairment,[19] but the significance of this action is unclear.

West Virginia's Workers' Compensation Division Health Advisory Panel has proposed that MCS not be compensable "due to absence of both physiologic basis for assessment and widely accepted etiologic cause in the workplace established by objective means."[20]

Despite this sound advice, many lawsuits have been based on allegations that chemical exposures cause disease by injuring the immune system. This notion is supported by a network of clinical ecologists and others who misinterpret laboratory data to support claims that virtually any symptom can be caused by exposure to almost anything. They testify that the immune system can become overactive (leading to numerous symptoms) or suppressed (leaving the individual at risk for infection, cancer, rheumatoid arthritis, and other diseases). The latter mechanism has been referred to as "chemical AIDS." Some cases involve people who are not physically ill but are afraid that low-dose exposure to environmental chemicals has affected their immune system and may make them susceptible to cancer or other diseases in the future.[21] Suits have even been brought alleging emotional distress over an allegedly toxic exposure.[22] The companies sued are not always large; small businesses have also been targets.

Legitimate cases exist where exposure to large or cumulative amounts of toxic chemicals has injured people. But in many of the cases described above, serious immune disorders are being alleged merely because laboratory testing has detected traces of a chemical in the body or has found a minor deviation from "normal" in some measure of immune function. Although no clinical injury is apparent, these plaintiffs are often said to have "chemical AIDS." Where many plaintiffs are involved, it would be prohibitively expensive for a defendant to examine all of them to obtain evidence to rebut the claims. Such "toxic tort" suits also carry a threat of punitive damages if the defendant loses. These factors may intimidate defendants into settling.[23]

In 1987, a Texas attorney began filing suit on behalf of 3,328 people who had worked at the Lone Star Steel Plant. The suit claimed the plant had infected them with "chemical AIDS," caused by a "toxic mushroom cloud" that "hovered ominously" for forty years over the company's property. The suit named 538 defendants, including companies that had supplied products used at the plant. *Forbes* magazine reported that when attorneys for the defense had attempted to find out about plaintiffs' alleged injuries, they were told that the information was not yet available—and their defense was stymied by a state court judge sympathetic to the plaintiffs. In 1995, the Texas Supreme Court ordered the plaintiffs to provide the requested information about the nature and the cause of their alleged illnesses, and a motion was made to dismiss 1,800 plaintiffs who had not answered basic discovery questions. The *Forbes* report states that about two hundred of the defendants and their insurance companies decided that settlement would be cheaper than legal fees and paid a total $70 million "over unproved charges for a nonexistent illness."[24]

In 1985, based on testimony by two clinical ecologists, a jury awarded a total of $6.2 million in compensatory damages and $43 million in punitive damages to thirty-two people who lived near a chemical plant in Sedalia, Missouri. This case and several others involving alleged illness due to chemical exposure have been analyzed by Peter W. Huber, an expert in liability law. In *Galileo's Revenge: Junk Science in the Courtroom,* Huber concluded that clinical ecologists are "perfectly adapted to modern-day testifying" because they are "adept at prevaricating, playing on credulity, scoring verbal points, forgetting inconvenient data, and dredging up convenient anecdotes."[25] Based on this case and others, the American Council on Science and Health has concluded:

MCS junk science is costing society millions of dollars. It is restricting people's lives in unnecessary ways and diverting them from effective medical treatment. It can cause enormous problems in the workplace and can cost people their jobs. It may burden the health-care system, severely tax the insurance industry, and wreak havoc with workers' compensation programs. It may also drive safe products from the market and make surviving products more expensive without improving their quality or safety.[26]

Fortunately, a 1993 U.S. Supreme Court decision has strengthened the ability of judges to exclude unscientific testimony. Rule 702 of the Federal Rules of Evidence states that expert testimony is admissible if it is relevant and the witness is qualified by knowledge, skill, experience, training, or education. In *Daubert* v. *Merrell Dow,* the court expanded this rule and stated:

In order to qualify as "scientific knowledge," an inference or assertion must be derived by the scientific method. . . .
　　Faced with a proffer of expert scientific testimony, then, the trial judge must determine at the outset . . . whether the expert is proposing to testify to (1) scientific knowledge that (2) will assist the trier of fact to understand or determine a fact in issue. This entails a preliminary assessment of whether the reasoning or methodology underlying the testimony is scientifically valid and of whether the reasoning or methodology properly can be applied to the facts in issue. . . .
　　Ordinarily, a key question to be answered in determining whether a theory or technique is scientific knowledge that will assist the trier of fact will be whether it can be (and has been) tested. . . .
　　Another pertinent consideration is whether the theory or technique has been subjected to peer review and publication. . . . Submission to the scrutiny of the scientific community is a component of "good science," in part because it increases the likelihood that substantive flaws in methodology will be detected. . . .
　　Widespread acceptance can be an important factor in ruling particular evidence admissible, and a known technique that has been able to attract only minimal support within the community may properly be viewed with skepticism.[27]

Timothy Kapshandy, an attorney who specializes in litigation involving scientific evidence, has noted:

Before the [*Daubert* decision] the validity of scientific evidence in all federal and most state courts was evaluated under a "general acceptance" standard. This generally meant that when controversial science was at issue, the proponent's expert would state that the methodology was "generally accepted," the opponent's expert would disagree, and the judge would let the jury decide. *Daubert* requires federal judges, not the jury, to evaluate the validity of the methodology and its applicability to the case. A number of state courts have adopted the *Daubert* guidelines.[28]

Appendix E of this book provides more of the text of the *Daubert* ruling. Appendix F summarizes thirty rulings adverse to clinical ecology theories and methodology. Although it is difficult to "keep score," Kapshandy believes that exclusion of dubious MCS-related testimony has increased. A state court judge recently stated that under *Daubert*, courts that have addressed the admissibility of the MCS diagnosis have generally rejected it.[29]

Some MCS proponents hope that shifting their terminology will prevent the courts from relying on previous rulings that MCS is not a valid diagnosis. As three attorneys recently noted:

Because MCS is controversial, many practitioners are now avoiding the more colorful names, and often refer to MCS as "not as a condition *per se*, but as a symptom complex resulting from a primary diagnosis, such as organic brain dysfunction or toxic encephalopathy."[30]

In one case, an appeals court reinstated the testimony of an MCS proponent who had carefully avoided calling the plaintiff's condition MCS.[31]

Many clinical ecologists have been inappropriately diagnosing "disorders of porphyrin metabolism" in a large percentage of their patients.[32] Porphyrias are metabolic disorders, usually hereditary, characterized by large amounts of porphyrin in the blood and urine. Their most frequent symptoms are hypersensitivity to sunlight, abdominal pain, constipation, diarrhea, and neurologic disturbances. Although the porphyrias are rare, MCS proponents claim that the majority of MCS patients have porphyrin abnormalities and that the same environmental substances can trigger both conditions.[33]

A recent article in *Our Toxic Times* said that diagnosing one of the porphyrias is advantageous because "they have a recognized diagnostic code" and "doctors who don't know about MCS or don't believe in it do believe in porphyria."[34] Another issue of the newsletter contains a "porphyria symptom check list" of about ninety "possible symptoms."[35] The Washington State Department of Labor and Industries and the Washington State Medical Association have issued an authoritative guide to diagnosing porphyrin disorders.[36] Expert reviewers have concluded that the proposed relationships between MCS and porphyrin disorders should be considered "speculative and unestablished" and do not justify using any measures that are appropriate for treating porphyrias.[37]

Several attorneys have advised their colleagues that "the ordinary process of litigation can be a health hazard for the client" because the paper generated by the litigation "may cause the client to become gravely ill." They warn:

> An MCS claimant alleged she had become ill from exposure to carbonless paper at work. During a hearing, counsel for the employer handed her a stack of carbonless paper for her to identify as the offending substance. Sometime after regaining consciousness, the client filed criminal assault charges and later a bar complaint against the attorney.

To minimize the alleged risks, they recommend (1) writing to clients in pencil, (2) airing photocopies for several days before sending them, (3) "testing" whether the client can tolerate rooms proposed for depositions, (4) requesting that no pens be used during depositions and that the court reporter dictate testimony into a mask rather than using an electric stenotype machine that contains ink, (5) asking participants not to wear perfume, recently polished shoes, or clothing that has recently been dry-cleaned or bleached, (6) conducting depositions by telephone, (7) obtaining documents well ahead of time so they can be aired out, and (8) using a videotaped deposition at trial so the client does not have to enter a courtroom where environmental conditions are difficult to control."[30]

The Bottom Line

The notion of chemical sensitivities has widespread appeal, even to those who do not believe themselves to be sufferers. Its appeal is enhanced by environmental worries; concerns about victimization; distrust of medicine, technology, and government; and growing interest in "alternative medicine."

However, "multiple chemical sensitivity" is not a legitimate diagnosis and is not caused by environmental chemicals. It is a phenomenon in which people misinterpret irritant or stress responses as "allergies" or "toxicities" and alter their behavior abnormally. Instead of testing their claims with well-designed research, its advocates are promoting them through publications, talk shows, support groups, lawsuits, and political maneuvering. Many are also part of a network of questionable legal actions alleging injuries by environmental chemicals.

Many people diagnosed with MCS suffer greatly and are very difficult to treat. Well-designed investigations suggest that most of them have a psychosomatic disorder in which they react to stress by developing multiple symptoms. If this is true—and we believe it is—clinical ecology patients run the risks of misdiagnosis, mistreatment, financial exploitation, and/or delay of proper medical and psychiatric care. In addition, insurance companies, employers, educational facilities, homeowners, other taxpayers, and ultimately all citizens are being burdened by dubious claims for disability and damages.

Recommendations

The MCS-related problems we describe in this book will not be simple to correct, but the following measures may help.

To state licensing boards
- Investigate clinical ecologists to determine whether the overall quality of their care is sufficient for them to remain in medical practice.

To scientific medical organizations
- Issue updated position papers on MCS and its associated trappings.
- Declare it unethical to administer diagnostic and treatment procedures that are unsubstantiated and lack a scientifically plausible rationale.
- Stop sponsoring dubious continuing education programs and withdraw accreditation from organizations that promote the concepts of clinical ecology or other unscientific medical practices.
- Press the American Academy of Otolaryngic Allergy to revoke its endorsement of unsubstantiated tests and procedures.

To physicians

- The terms MCS, EI, and the like should be abandoned and replaced by a diagnostic term that does not imply an unsubstantiated cause.
- Remember that patients with multiple symptoms are suffering. Try to explain how stress often leads to symptoms, and to persuade them to seek mental help.

To psychiatrists, psychologists, and other mental health workers

- Do not reinforce unsubstantiated beliefs about MCS.
- Aim to establish trust and rapport. Then help patients manage their symptoms, cope with their limitations, and restructure their beliefs about their health.

To clinical ecologists

- Set up genuine protocols so that your data can be tabulated and put in publishable form.
- Abandon provocation-neutralization and other questionable tests unless their value is repeatedly demonstrated by well designed double-blind studies.
- Abandon the other trappings of quackery, such as useless dietary supplements, homeopathic products, and sauna "detoxification" or "purification."

To manufacturers

- Industries at risk, including insurance companies, food and chemical manufacturers, the cosmetics industry, and employers, should provide independently administered funds to help solve MCS-related problems.
- Some of the money should be used for research. Priority should be given to double-blind, placebo-controlled studies to determine whether patients' symptoms are actually caused by chemical sensitivity. At present, few facilities in the United States can perform such testing.
- Other money should be used to maintain a clearinghouse for information on the scientific, legal, and political issues. The information should include scientific reports, legal case reports, and prior testimony by potential expert witnesses.

To judges

- Use the criteria set forth in the *Daubert* case to exclude unhelpful testimony.

To legislators
- Don't permit "alternative" practitioners to practice under standards lower than those by which science-based practitioners are judged.
- Don't legislate money for MCS-related research that has no practical value.
- Don't permit MCS claimants to be compensated under the Americans with Disability Act for other than psychiatric reasons.
- Don't enact laws that enable MCS patients to infringe on the rights of others.

To the National Institute of Environmental Health Sciences
- Stop distributing literature which suggests that MCS is a clearly defined disease entity caused by exposure to environmental chemicals.

To patients and their families
- Remember that MCS is a label, not a disease. The symptoms associated with the MCS diagnosis are likely to be bodily reactions to stress. Don't seek treatment with a clinical ecologist. Go instead to a mental health practitioner who can explore how the symptoms arise and what can be done to overcome them.
- If a family member falls under the spell of a clinical ecologist, act quickly to protect yourself. Don't permit your love to lead you to financial ruin.

To educators
- Do not agree to provide "safe rooms," home tutoring, or other special accommodations for children with MCS, because these accommodations send false messages to children about their health status.

To researchers
- Set up inpatient/outpatient treatment units that offer treatment under scientifically sound protocols.
- Limit other research to hypotheses that are plausible, testable, and likely to produce information that is medically useful or can help courts and regulatory agencies make equitable decisions.

To insurance companies
- Check your policies to be sure that the nonstandard diagnostic and treatment methods used by clinical ecologists are excluded. Be alert to the possibility that some patients may be improperly reported as having porphyria or a yeast infection.

To the news media

- Don't glorify MCS patients. Articles that could stimulate readers to consult clinical ecologists have great potential for harm. Public information should be based on established fact, not speculation.

References

1. The American Academy of Environmental Medicine's 1996–1997 membership directory lists 429 individuals, about 75% of whom are medical or osteopathic physicians practicing in the United States.
2. Travers B, editor. Encyclopedia of Medical Agencies and Organizations, Seventh Edition, 1998. Detroit: Gale Research, 1997.
3. 1989 position statements of the Academy of Otolaryngic Allergy (AAOA).
4. Kroll-Smith S, Floyd HH. Bodies in Protest: Environmental Illness and the Struggle over Medical Knowledge. New York: New York University Press, 1997.
5. Hospitality Plus: The HEAL Travel Guide. Atlanta: Human Ecology Action League, 1996.
6. Wilson C. Welcome to CINN. White Sulfur Springs, Mont.: Chemical Injury Information Network, 1994.
7. Wilson C. MCS advocates form the Chemical Injury Council. Our Toxic Times 7(10):16–17, 1996.
8. Adams JM. Perfume industry targeted by anti-fragrance activists. Sacramento Bee, Oct. 25, 1994.
9. Perfume protest at Fairmont Hotel. Mask-wearing demonstrators say scents make them sick. San Francisco Chronicle, Oct. 25, 1994:A16.
10. Multiple chemical sensitivity. National Institute of Environmental Health Sciences, undated flyer distributed in 1997.
11. Americans with Disabilities Act of 1990, Public law 101-366; USC 12101 et seq., 1990.
12. Dolin LH. How to marshal the power of the Americans with Disabilities Act to minimize your company's exposure to liability to individuals seeking accommodations for "multiple chemical sensitivity disabilities." Regulatory Toxicology and Pharmacology 24:S168–181, 1996.
13. Souder W. A fragrance violation? Washington Post, Dec. 11, 1994:F1, F4.
14. Raising a chemically sensitive child. Part 2: School, camp, and college. The Human Ecologist 72:9–12, 1996.
15. Appleby J. Built to be bare: In Marin County, a HUD-backed haven for the chemically sensitive. Washington Post, March 2, 1995:8–11.
16. Adams JM. Nontoxic home project faulted. Chemically sensitive tenants say house is no refuge. Dallas Morning News, March 12, 1995.
17. Gots RE. State of the science review: Multiple chemical sensitivities. North Bethesda, Md.: Environmental Sensitivities Research Institute, 1995.

18. Custer WV. Multiple chemical sensitivity syndrome: The wavering influence of the courts on public policy. Regulatory Toxicology and Pharmacology 24:S182–187, 1996.

19. Goodwin KL. Defendant's supplemental memorandum, Oct. 31, 1997. Creamer *v.* Sullivan. U.S. District Court for the District of Massachusetts, Civil Action No. 97-30040-KPN.

20. Proposed Legislative Rule. Multiple Chemical Sensitivity, Series 28, §85-28-2 through §85-28-7, West Virginia Worker's Compensation Division, 1997.

21. Brown RS, Lees-Haley PR. Fear of future illness: Chemical AIDS and cancerphobia: A review. Psychological Reports 71:187–207, 1992.

22. Bisbing SB. Cancerphobia and related cases: Review of case law. The Personal Injury Law Defense Bulletin, Issue No. 5, Feb.1989:2.

23. Willmore RL. In fear of cancerphobia. Defense Counsel Journal 56:50–57, 1989.

24. Adams S. The 1000-year lawsuit. Forbes 158(17):166–172, 1996.

25. Huber PW: Galileo's Revenge: Junk Science in the Courtroom. New York: Basic Books, 1991.

26. Orme TW, Benedetti P. Multiple Chemical Sensitivity. New York: American Council on Science and Health, 1993.

27. Daubert v. Merrell Dow Pharmaceuticals, Inc. 113 S. Ct. 2786 (U.S. 1993).

28. Kapshandy T. The changing view of science by courts. Presented at the Second Annual Environmental Medicine Conference, Aspen Colorado, Sept. 9, 1995.

29. Defense verdict for school district on former student's pesticide exposure claims. Mealey's Emerging Toxic Torts 5(22):4–5, 1997.

30. Lieberman MS, Di Muro BJ, Boyd JB. Multiple chemical sensitivity: An emerging area of law. Trial, July 1995:22–33.

31. Hottinger v. Truegreen Corp, 665 N.E. 2nd 293, Ind. Ct. App. 1996.

32. Wilson C. Porphyrinopathies in the MCS community. Our Toxic Times 7(3):1–4, 1996.

33. Morton W. Chronic porphyrias' role in MCS. Our Toxic Times 6(8):22–24, 1995.

34. Wilson C. Hallmark feature of MCS and porphyria. Our Toxic Times 7(10):1–8, 1996.

35. Porphyria symptom check list. Our Toxic Times 7(6):20–21, 1996.

36. Collaborative guidelines on the diagnosis of porphyria and related conditions. Olympia, Wa.: Washington State Department of Labor and Industries, Oct. 18, 1995.

37. Daniell WE and others. Environmental chemical exposures and disturbances of heme synthesis. Environmental Health Perspectives 105(Suppl 1):37–53, 1997.

5

The "Candidiasis" Epidemic

Candida albicans (sometimes referred to as monilia) is a fungus normally present on the skin and in the mouth, intestinal tract, and vagina. Under certain conditions, it can multiply and infect the surface of the skin or mucous membranes. Such infections are usually minor, but serious and deeper infections can occur in patients whose resistance has been weakened by immunosuppressant drugs and serious illnesses such as AIDS. However, some practitioners claim that even when clinical signs of infection are absent, yeast-related problems can cause or trigger multiple symptoms such as fatigue, irritability, constipation, diarrhea, abdominal bloating, mood swings, depression, anxiety, dizziness, unexpected weight gain, difficulty in concentrating, muscle and joint pain, cravings for sugar or alcoholic beverages, psoriasis, hives, respiratory and ear problems, menstrual problems, infertility, impotence, bladder infections, prostate inflammation, and "feeling bad all over." The list of symptoms is similar to that of multiple chemical sensitivity (MCS).

Far-Fetched Claims

According to its promoters, one out of three Americans suffers from yeast-related illness, which proponents refer to as chronic candidiasis, candidiasis hypersensitivity, Candida-related complex, the yeast syndrome, yeast allergy, yeast overgrowth, or simply "Candida" or "yeast problem." Many clinical ecologists view this alleged problem as an underlying cause of MCS. It is also touted as an important factor in AIDS, rheumatoid arthritis, multiple sclerosis, and schizophrenia, as well as "hypoglycemia," "mercury-amalgam toxicity," and at least twenty other conditions. In recent years, proponents have suggested that chronic fatigue syndrome and Candida infections are closely related. One states that "chronic fatigue syndrome is Candida under a different name."[1] In this book, we use the term "candidiasis hypersensitivity" in quotation marks to indicate that neither infection nor actual sensitivity is present.

The leading promoters of "candidiasis hypersensitivity" have been C. Orian Truss, M.D., of Birmingham, Alabama; William G. Crook, M.D., of Jackson, Tennessee; and John Parks Trowbridge, M.D., of Humble, Texas. Truss put forth his concepts with a series of articles that began in 1978 in the *Journal of Orthomolecular Psychiatry*, an offbeat publication that caters to physicians who prescribe large amounts of vitamins to emotionally disturbed patients. In 1982, he self-published a book called *The Missing Diagnosis*, which included the following "typical clinical picture":

> A woman between puberty and menopause who has begun having vaginal symptoms (discharge, itching or both) and/or bowel symptoms (constipation or diarrhea, excess "gas," abdominal distention and discomfort), abnormalities of the menstrual cycle or flow, absent or diminished libido, and a personality change characterized by abnormal emotions (depression, extreme irritability, anxiety, crying), deterioration in intellectual function (concentration, memory, reasoning), and a destructive loss of self-confidence so severe that it may result in her inability to cope with even the simplest problem.[2]

Crook states that he began treating and communicating about yeast problems in 1979 after reading one of Truss's papers. In 1983, he published the first edition of his book *The Yeast Connection*,[3] which he says was inspired by a television appearance that drew 7,300 requests for further information. Two years later, he established the International Health Foundation to help respond to the requests he kept generating. The foundation's goals were to "work to obtain credibility for the relationship of Candida albicans to a diverse group of health disorders" and "helping children with repeated ear infections, hyperactivity, attention deficits and related behavior and learning problems." (Crook also espoused a variety of unconventional theories about allergies being at the root of these problems.) During the early 1990s, a booklet describing these goals listed Tipper Gore as a member of the foundation's thirty-three-person advisory board.[4] Mrs. Gore's husband—Al Gore—was subsequently elected U.S. Vice President.

The Yeast Connection states: "If a careful check-up doesn't reveal the cause for your symptoms, and your medical history [as described in his book] is typical, it's possible or even probable that your health problems are yeast-connected." The book also states that tests such as cultures don't help much in diagnosis because "Candida germs live in every person's body. . . . Therefore the diagnosis is suspected from the patient's history and confirmed by his response to treatment."

Crook claims that the problem arises because "antibiotics kill 'friendly germs' while they're killing enemies, and when friendly germs are knocked out, yeast germs multiply. Diets rich in carbohydrates and yeasts, birth control pills, cortisone and other drugs also stimulate yeast growth." He also claims that the yeasts produce toxins that weaken the immune system, which is also adversely affected by nutritional deficiencies, sugar consumption, and exposure to environmental molds and chemicals. To correct these alleged problems, he prescribes allergenic extracts, antifungal drugs, vitamin and mineral supplements, and diets that avoid refined carbohydrates, processed foods, and (initially) fruits and milk.

Crook's concepts are a mixture of fact and fancy. It is correct that antibiotics, birth control pills, and certain other drugs can stimulate overgrowth of yeasts, most commonly in the vagina. However, a yeast problem should not be diagnosed without definite clinical signs of an infection. The signs of a local infection, for example, can include itching, soreness, rash, and a discharge. If an infection is present, antibiotic treatment makes sense. However, the rest of Crook's recommendations are senseless whether an infection is present or not.

Dubious Diagnostic Questionnaires

The Yeast Connection contains a seventy-item questionnaire and score sheet to determine how likely it is that health problems are yeast-connected. Trowbridge's book *The Yeast Syndrome* groups two hundred symptoms according to ten "body systems" and scores those that are present from 1 to 3, depending on their frequency. According to Trowbridge:

> Any group in which you score fifteen points or more, you must consider that candidiasis might be causing problems in that body system. Any group in which you score ten to fourteen points, you should consider that candidiasis possibly contributes to problems in that body system. Any group in which you score less than ten points but you've marked several answers with the number 3 or 2, consider that candidiasis may be weakening that body system. In fact, pay attention to any individual "3" response. This higher number will alert your physician to check more closely the particular body tissue, organ, or system for effects of yeast infestation or other disturbance to body function.[5]

Shorter questionnaires have appeared in magazine articles, ads for products sold through health food stores, and flyers used by chiropractors.

In 1986, an article in *Redbook* magazine asked readers whether they (1) had ever taken antibiotics on a frequent basis; (2) had ever been troubled by premenstrual tension, abdominal pain, or loss of sexual interest; (4) craved sugar, breads, or alcoholic beverages; (3) had recurrent digestive problems; (5) got moderate to severe symptoms when exposed to tobacco smoke; (6) experienced fatigue, depression, poor memory, or nervous tension; (7) were bothered by hives, psoriasis, or other chronic skin rashes; (8) had ever taken birth control pills; (9) were bothered by headaches; or (10) felt bad all over without any apparent cause. According to the article, "If you have three or four 'yes' answers, yeast possibly plays a role in causing your symptoms. If you have five or six 'yes' answers, yeast probably plays a role in causing your symptoms. If you have seven or more 'yes' answers, your symptoms are almost certainly yeast-connected."[6] The article's author was said to be "on her way to recovery" from a debilitating case of "the yeast syndrome."

Crook's book and frequent television appearances enabled many others to take advantage of the situation. Several other books have been published, and many manufacturers market "yeast-free" dietary supplements which presumably are "safer" than ordinary ones. Health-food-industry manufacturers, including several that market through chiropractors, have also offered such products as *Candi-Care, Candida-Guard, Candida Cleanse, Candistat, Cantrol, Yeast Fighters, Yeast Guard, Yeastop, Yeasterol,* and *Yeast•Trol.*

Before the *Redbook* article was published, *Cantrol*'s manufacturer notified retailers that an ad in the same issue would "specifically instruct the consumer to go to their local health food store to purchase *Cantrol*." The ad contained a toll-free number for ordering the product or obtaining further information. According to a company official, more than 100,000 people responded.[8]

Severe Criticism

The American Academy of Allergy, Asthma and Immunology has strongly criticized the concept of "candidiasis hypersensitivity syndrome" and the diagnostic and treatment approaches its proponents use. AAAAI's position statement concludes: (1) the concept of candidiasis hypersensitivity is speculative and unproven; (2) its basic elements would apply to almost all sick patients at some time because its supposed symptoms are essentially universal; (3) overuse of oral antifungal agents could lead to the development of resistant germs that could menace others; (4) adverse effects of oral antifungal agents are rare, but some inevitably will occur; and (5) neither patients nor doctors can determine effectiveness (as opposed to coincidence) without controlled trials. Because allergic symptoms can be influenced by many factors, including emotions, experiments must be designed to separate the effects of the procedure being tested from the effects of other factors.[9] Appendix B contains the full text of this report. Several years ago, Crook told Dr. Stephen Barrett that he had no intention of conducting a controlled test because he was "a clinician, not a researcher."

The antifungal drug most often prescribed by proponents of "candidiasis hypersensitivity" is nystatin (*Mycostatin, Nilstat*), which seldom has significant side effects. However, they also prescribe ketoconazole (*Nizoral*), which has an incidence of liver toxicity (hepatitis) of about 1 in 10,000. The liver injury usually reverses when the drug is discontinued, but ketoconazole has been responsible for several deaths. For this reason it should be prescribed only for serious infections. Both of these drugs are expensive.[10] In a double-blind trial, the antifungal drug nystatin did no better than a placebo in relieving systemic or psychologic symptoms of patients said to have "candidiasis hypersensitivity syndrome."[11]

Problems Reported

In 1986, two doctors from Loyola University Stritch School of Medicine reported seeing four young women whose nonspecific complaints included chronic fatigue, anxiety, and depression. All four mistakenly believed they had disseminated candidiasis and were taking nystatin or ketoconazole, which had been prescribed by their family physicians. All had read *The Yeast Connection* and had carried the book into the office during their visits. One patient on ketoconazole had hepatitis, which resolved when the drug was stopped.[12]

Worse yet, a case has been reported of a child with a severe case of disseminated candidiasis who had been seen by a "Candida doctor" and given inadequate treatment. The report concluded that "the advice of yeast connection advocates may be inappropriate even for illnesses in which Candida is implicated."[13]

Perhaps the saddest report was a letter in a health-food magazine from a woman appealing for help and encouragement. She said that a clinical ecologist had been treating her for allergies and Candida for four years, that initial tests showed she "was allergic to all foods" as well as to numerous chemicals and inhalants, and that so far nothing had helped.

In 1990, "Inside Edition" aired two segments vilifying Stuart Berger, M.D., a Park Avenue "diet doctor" who wrote *Dr. Berger's Immune Power Diet* and *What Your Doctor Didn't Learn in Medical School.* During the first program, a reporter described what happened when she visited Berger complaining of fatigue. So did a prominent New York allergist who consulted Berger with a similar complaint. Both noted that their contact with him lasted about two minutes, included no physical examination, and culminated with diagnoses of chronic fatigue syndrome and yeast allergy. The reporter's cost was $845 for the first visit, with an estimated total of about $1,500 through the third visit. A former patient described a similar experience which had cost over $1,000. And a former employee said that Berger ordered his employees to indicate on blood test reports that every patient was allergic to wheat, dairy products, eggs, and yeast.

The reporter's visit had been filmed with a hidden camera. When Berger found out about this, he obtained a court order stopping "Inside Edition" from showing the tape during the initial program. But two weeks later, after the U.S. Supreme Court sided with the producers, the tape was shown. During the interim, complaints were received from more than a hundred former patients and employees.

In 1985, *Dr. Berger's Immune Power Diet* had become an overnight best seller following Berger's appearance on the "Donahue" show. The book claimed that being overweight and numerous other health problems are the result of an "immune hypersensitivity response" to common foods, and that "detoxification" and weight loss followed by dietary supplements can tune and strengthen the immune system. There is no scientific evidence to support these claims.

Government Actions

Under federal law, any product intended for the prevention or treatment of disease is a drug, and it is illegal to market new drugs that do not have FDA approval. In 1989, the FDA's Health Fraud Branch issued instructions and a sample regulatory letter indicating that it was illegal to market vitamin products intended for treating yeast infections.

During 1988, the FDA initiated a seizure of *Yeastop*, a vitamin concoction claimed to be effective against yeast microorganisms that have become "overgrown" or "out of control." The manufacturer, Nature's Herbs, of Orem, Utah, claimed that the product was a "dietary supplement." But the FDA charged that the therapeutic claims on its label made it an illegal drug. In 1990, a federal judge ruled that *Yeastop* was a drug and ordered Nature's Herbs to pay for its destruction and for other court costs and fees. The FDA also seized a supply of *Cantrol* from its manufacturer, Nature's Way, of Springville, Utah.

In 1989, Great Earth International, the nation's second largest health food store chain, agreed to pay $100,000 in penalties plus $9,520 in costs to settle charges filed in 1987 by the Orange County (California) District Attorney. The case involved advertising claims for *Yeasterol* ("to control . . . Candida albicans, a troublesome yeast") and several other products. Without admitting wrongdoing, the company signed a consent agreement pledging to refrain from marketing products that are misbranded or are unapproved new drugs.

In 1990, Nature's Way and its president, Kenneth Murdock, settled a Federal Trade Commission complaint by signing a consent agreement to stop making unsubstantiated claims that *Cantrol* is helpful against yeast infections caused by *Candida albicans*. The product, a conglomeration of capsules containing acidophilus, evening primrose oil, vitamin E, linseed oil, caprylic acid, pau d'arco, and several other substances, was promoted with a self-test based on common symptoms the manufacturer claimed were associated with yeast problems. The FTC

Take the Yeast Test.

Do you have a yeast problem? Here's what it is and how to fight it.

We call the type of yeast normally found in our bodies "Candida colonies." Normally they are harmless. However, they can sometimes grow rapidly due to a variety of conditions. When this happens they are no longer friendly microorganisms, but have developed into a "Candida albicans" problem. Worse, they have an adverse effect on our health.

Nature's Way, the makers of Cantrol™, a total nutritional plan designed to help control Candida albicans, has developed a simple test to help you determine if you have a yeast problem.*

Y N
1. Do you feel tired most of the time?
2. Do you suffer from intestinal gas, abdominal bloating or discomfort?
3. Do you crave sugar, bread, beer or other alcoholic beverages?
4. Are you bothered by constipation, diarrhea, or alternating constipation and diarrhea?
5. Do you suffer from mood swings or depression?
6. Are you often irritable, easily angered, anxious or nervous?
7. Do you have trouble thinking clearly, suffer occasional memory losses or have difficulty concentrating?
8. Are you ever dizzy or lightheaded?
9. Do you have muscle aches or stiffness with normal activity?
10. Have you had an unexpected weight gain without a change in diet?
11. Are you bothered by itching or burning of the vagina or prostate or a loss of sexual desire?
12. Have you ever taken antibiotics?
13. Are you currently or have you ever used birth control pills?
14. Have you ever taken steroid drugs, such as cortisone?

*This quiz is provided for general information only and is not intended to be used for self-diagnosis without the advice and examination of a qualified health professional. Some of the symptoms could indicate a more serious condition which could require the assistance of a health professional.

If you answered 6 or more questions with a "yes," you may have a yeast problem. Read about how Cantrol can help.

Portion of a *Cantrol* ad from the May1986 issue of *Let's Live* magazine. The ad and one for *The Yeast Connection* were adjacent to an article recommending dietary supplements for treating candidiasis.

charged that the test was not valid for this purpose. The company also agreed to pay $30,000 to the National Institutes of Health to support research on yeast infections.

These government actions have driven most of the "anti-Candida" concoctions from the marketplace and stopped their direct promotion to the public. However, the ingredients of these products are still marketed individually as "dietary supplements" and practitioners still prescribe them to their patients.

In 1990, the New Jersey State Attorney General secured consent agreements barring Linda Choi, M.D., and Pruyakant Doshi, M.D., from diagnosing and treating "Candida albicans overgrowth syndrome." Both were assessed $3,000 for investigative costs and had their medical license placed on probation for one year. Among other things, investigation by the State medical board had concluded that "Candida albicans overgrowth" was not generally recognized as a clinical entity and had not been established as the cause of the conditions the doctors treated. We believe that doctors who diagnose nonexistent "yeast problems" should have their licenses revoked.

References

1. Yeast-related illness: Three interviews. The Human Ecologist, Winter 1992, pp. 9–11.
2. Truss CO. The Missing Diagnosis. Birmingham: The Missing Diagnosis, Inc., 1983.
3. Crook, WG. The Yeast Connection—A Medical Breakthrough. Jackson, Tenn.: Professional Books, 1983, 1984, 1986.
4. Crook W. There Are Better Ways to Help These Children (booklet). Jackson, Tenn.: International Health Foundation, undated, circa 1991.
5. Trowbridge JP, Walker M. The Yeast Syndrome: How to Help Your Doctor and Identify and Treat the Real Cause of Your Yeast-Related Illness. New York: Bantam Books, 1986.
6. Thomas DC. The newest mystery illness. Redbook 166:120–121, 152–153, April 1986.
7. Barrett S, Herbert V. The Vitamin Pushers: How the "Health Food" Industry Is Selling America a Bill of Goods. Amherst, N.Y.: Prometheus Books, 1994.
8. Levin LB. Controlling yeast overgrowth—Consumer concern prompts the industry to respond with new products and information. Natural Foods Merchandiser 9(1):32, 34–35, 1987.

9. Anderson JA and others. Position statement on candidiasis hypersensitivity. Journal of Allergy and Clinical Immunology 78:271–273, 1986.
10. Tabor E. Potential toxicity of ketoconazole. Journal of Infectious Disease 152:233, 1985.
11. Dismukes W and others. A randomized double-blind trial of nystatin therapy for the candidiasis hypersensitivity syndrome. New England Journal of Medicine 323:1717–1723, 1990.
12. Quinn JP and others. Ketoconazole and the yeast connection. JAMA 255:3250, 1986.
13. Haas A and others. The "Yeast Connection" meets chronic mucocutaneous candidiasis. New England Journal of Medicine 314:854–855, 1986.

6

Confusion about "Sick Buildings"

Like MCS, sick building syndrome (SBS) is not a disease. It is a phenomenon in which many people who work in the same building develop symptoms with no apparent cause. Like MCS, the nature of SBS is elusive, its causes are ill-defined, and attempts to solve it have proven expensive and time-consuming.

The idea that buildings can be dangerous received massive publicity in 1976 when a mysterious lung ailment killed twenty-nine people who attended an American Legion convention at the Bellevue-Stratford Hotel in Philadelphia. Careful sleuthing ultimately identified the culprit as a bacterium that multiplied in the air-conditioning system and was released into the building.[1,2] A new affliction (Legionnaires' disease) was diagnosed, and the cause was clearly identified. The building was indeed hazardous.

Concern about indoor air increased with the issue of urea-formaldehyde foam insulation. In the mid-1970s, when energy conservation was paramount, this product was touted as a major energy-saving device. As a result, it was sprayed into the walls of homes throughout the country until health complaints and lawsuits erupted. The complaints involved irritant effects as well as serious illnesses. How many of these problems were actually caused by chemical emissions from the foam is unclear. Nevertheless, the Consumer Product Safety Commission banned its use and furthered the perception that noxious chemicals emitted from energy-efficient, well-insulated buildings are a threat to health.

Since the early 1980s, the term "sick building syndrome" has been used to describe multiple subjective complaints reported by workers in modern office buildings. The most frequent symptoms are irritation of the eyes, nose, and throat. Other common complaints are headache, confusion, fatigue, difficulty concentrating, and respiratory distress. Less common are vocal cord dysfunction, gastrointestinal complaints, fainting, and rashes. Many people think that airborne contaminants are responsible for these symptoms.

Like MCS, SBS is a focus of considerable controversy. Consider the following events.

• In 1985, a Bell South facility in Orange County, California, had a sudden outbreak of fainting episodes. The building was evacuated, hazardous-material and fire-department teams combed the building seeking a cause, and affected workers were taken to local hospitals for treatment. Examinations of both the building and the workers did not reveal any noxious chemicals or measurable physical damage to the workers. Ultimately, it was determined that a disgruntled employee had started a rumor about a dangerous chemical loose in the building.

• In the early 1990s, fifteen employees of an accounting firm in Los Angeles sued the developer of their building, claiming that a variety of ailments were related to working in the building. No physical basis could be found to connect their complaints to any characteristic of the building. Yet the case was settled out-of-court for several million dollars.

• During the same time period, the Martin County Courthouse in Florida was the site of daily health complaints by a significant portion of its employee-occupants. Millions of dollars were spent remediating the new courthouse — more than its original cost. The purpose of remediation was to solve water-seepage problems that resulted in mold growth. The mold was considered to be the cause of employee health complaints. The workers' diagnoses ranged from mold-related asthma and lung allergies to depression and other psychogenic symptoms. No conclusive link between the presence of mold and reported symptoms was ever established. Yet the county sued the builder and won a $14.2 million judgment. In a similar case, officials from Polk County, Florida, sued the insurance company that had guaranteed the work of the courthouse builder and won a $34 million judgment. In another sick building controversy, officials in DuPage County, Illinois, won a $21,000 judgment against the building's developer but spent $2.4 million on legal fees.

• In 1995, FBI agents in Fort Lauderdale, Florida, filed a suit claiming that their health problems were associated with the federal courthouse. County officials have spent nearly $1 million on studies and repairs to their courthouse following complaints of workers.

• In 1996, workers in a Chicago department store complained that bad air in their building had made them ill, even though their doctors had diagnosed their symptoms as psychosomatic or stress-related. Rather than acknowledge that their problems had a psychological component, the workers filed suit.

• In April 1996, the U.S. Department of Transportation announced a sick-building problem and indicated that 5,500 employees could be affected.

• In July 1997, four federal unions demanded new federal guidelines for dealing with sick building syndrome. The unions identified thirty federal buildings nationwide where workers' alleged illness related to poor air quality. The reported symptoms included headaches, nausea, eye and skin irritation, sinus problems, coughing, and other respiratory problems.

Health complaints associated with buildings can be placed into two main categories: building-related diseases and sick building syndrome.[3] The classification depends on whether a specific disease and a causal agent can be identified. The key question for evaluating these situations is whether the cause of the problem is physical (a noxious chemical or an infectious agent) or psychological.

Building-Related Diseases (BRDs)

Building-related diseases are caused by identifiable contaminants of indoor air. The problems can range from mild to severe.[4,5] Certain bacteria and molds commonly found in heating and air-conditioning systems can cause respiratory problems. Molds, for example, can produce mild allergic conditions such as hay fever, as well as serious diseases such as asthma or hypersensitivity pneumonia. Common viral illnesses—colds and influenza—can also spread through ventilation systems. When many members of a workforce become ill through this means, that is also classifiable as BRD. Sometimes a specific environmental contributor can be identified. For example, a study of army recruits living in "leaky" barracks versus those living in "tight," more energy-efficient barracks found that the latter group had a higher frequency of colds.[6] It is certainly reasonable to assume that poor ventilation will help respiratory viruses spread throughout a building.

To classify an outbreak as a BRD, there must be clear evidence that a causal agent is present in the building. Moreover, the disease must be a specific condition that can be observed and quantified, not simply a set of symptoms or general complaints. It could be a fatal respiratory illness, as occurred in the 1976 Legionnaires' disease outbreak. It could be an epidemic of influenza that passes through a workforce. It could be occupation-related asthma verified by immunologic tests, bacterial cultures, or measurable levels of contaminants found in a building's ventilation system.

Sick Building Syndrome (SBS)

The term "sick building syndrome" has been applied to situations in which at least 20 percent of a workforce has varied symptoms with no demonstrable external cause.[7-9] SBS differs from BRD because a specific cause generally can not be identified; or, if one is determined, a link between the cause and symptoms remains unclear. In essence, SBS is a descriptive term indicating that occupants of a building are not feeling well. The term does not explain why their symptoms occur, but only that they may be related to working in a specific building.

The development of SBS usually follows three stages: (1) an underlying stressor is present, which can be physiologic or psychologic; (2) a trigger event leads employees to conclude that their symptoms may be related to the workplace environment; and (3) a crisis of concern develops.

Sometimes symptoms arise because employees are under stress and develop headaches and other symptoms. Poor ventilation, described as "stuffy air," can be a cause that is identified by finding elevated carbon dioxide levels in the air. The symptoms can also result from a specific chemical that causes irritant effects but produces no physical findings in employees. Some studies have concluded that environmental factors such as lighting and volatile organic compounds were involved. All of these situations and several others have been closely studied.[10-16]

Unfortunately, the large variety of potential causes makes investigation of cause-and-effect relationships difficult.[17] Researchers at the University of California at Davis have noted:

> Many of the symptoms that people attribute to sick building syndrome (SBS) or building-related illness, such as headaches, dizziness, fatigue, nausea, cough, and eye irritation, are subjective, and studies often fail to take into account other possible causes that may be inherent in the subjects, such as sinusitis, hyperventilation syndrome, or psychosomatic illness. Unfortunately, most clinical studies on SBS pay little attention to the preexisting conditions that a subject may have and discount the possibility that the inciting agent does not cause symptoms, but merely exacerbates a preexisting condition. Moreover, they offer no information about the nature of the mechanisms of action or pathophysiological relationships. Clearly, further studies are necessary to further explain the complexity of complaints that currently exist. Indeed, SBS might properly be paraphrased as, "What is it?—if it is!"[18]

These researchers are among those who argue—correctly, we believe—that the term "sick building syndrome" should be abandoned because it perpetuates a false belief that persistent generalized symptoms are likely to have poor indoor-air quality as their cause.[19]

Elusive Causes

Because SBS is associated with nonspecific symptoms and uses subjective questionnaires for its identification, toxic and psychogenic factors may be difficult to separate.[20,21] Causative factors can include high outdoor pollen count, high prevalence of a viral illness in the community, job stress, worker dissatisfaction, computer-related discomfort, use of contact lenses, and variations in the frequency of reporting complaints.[22-24]

The number of complaints is not sufficient evidence that air quality is the culprit. Nor do the symptoms themselves establish the cause. Reported SBS symptoms typically vary from person to person and from building to building and are sufficiently nonspecific to obscure whether they have a common cause. Moreover, consistent physical findings are absent. (If they were present, the problem would be a BRD.) Nonetheless, there is a popular belief that SBS does exist.

The difficulty of pinning down building-related causes for physical complaints is illustrated by a study comparing groups of people in two buildings in Washington, D.C.[25] One group complained of symptoms that they related to poor indoor air quality. The other group was selected from a nearby building whose workers had not complained. Both groups were given symptom questionnaires. Forty percent of those in the allegedly "sick building" returned the questionnaires, whereas 25 percent in the control "healthy building" returned theirs. The symptoms reported were identical for responders in both groups—with headaches and sinus problems predominating. It is unclear whether the greater frequency of response from those working in the "sick building" (40 percent versus 25 percent) was related to real physical problems caused by bad air or to a perception that the building air posed a health hazard.

Another recently published study found that large percentages of people in nonproblem buildings had symptoms.[26] Four different buildings were included, three located in a semi-urban environment and an older building located in a dense urban area. Using specified criteria, the EPA's Indoor Air Building Assessment Survey and Evaluation Program had classified them nonproblem buildings. Three of the four buildings had operable windows. Fifty-five percent of the 646 respondents reported recent symptoms that affected their eyes, nose, or throat and improved when away from work. Over half were upper respiratory in nature and occurred one to three times a week. Forty-eight percent reported central nervous system symptoms. Statistical analysis indicated the following:

- The rates of reporting symptoms were highest in two buildings with operable windows.

- The symptoms were not related to environmental concentrations of aldehydes, carbon dioxide, or humidity or to the presence of bacteria.

- Upper respiratory symptoms were related to perceptions of workstation cleanliness, comfort, privacy, use of contact lenses, and satisfaction with the workstation.

- For central nervous system symptoms, gender differences represented the strongest association, with women reporting 2.6 times as many problems as men reported.

- Lower respiratory symptoms (chest tightness, wheezing, and shortness of breath) were associated with perceptions of limited air movement, odors, and job stress.

- The symptoms were statistically related to the presence of volatile compounds, dust, noise and illumination.

These findings indicate that the symptoms associated with SBS are common complaints found in the population-at-large. Basic psychologic studies have found that people who perceive a health threat are more likely to respond to symptom questionnaires than those who do not.[27-30]

Some people argue that energy-efficient construction results in the accumulation of contaminants that, in less efficient buildings, would wind up outdoors. While it is clear that modern buildings have less communication with outdoor air, it is not clear that indoor air today is worse than it used to be. For example, in this country, smoking in the workplace is often prohibited. Before these bans, conference rooms and offices often were filled with cigarette and even cigar smoke (hence the expression "smoke-filled rooms"). What could be more contaminating than the hundreds of irritating chemicals emitted by tobacco smoke? That indoor air environment was far more contaminated than that of today's workplaces in which minuscule amounts of unseen and often unsmelled chemicals have become the focus of intense concern.

As reports of indoor air problems intensify, so will psychological factors contributing to symptom development. In many situations, the only way to be sure whether an airborne chemical is the culprit would be through controlled, blinded studies in which exposure to air constituents are varied without the knowledge of the test subject. The few studies of this type done so far have found little relationship between air-exchange rates, contaminant levels, and symptoms.

Measurements Can Mislead

The science of measurement has advanced rapidly, enabling us to detect indoor air contaminants at extremely low levels (parts per quadrillion). This ability enables detection of quantities too small to have physiologic or toxicologic significance. Surveys—whether conducted in homes, businesses, or outdoors—may detect hundreds of airborne chemicals and microorganisms that have no practical significance.

A 1989 report by the World Health Organization (WHO) Committee on Indoor Air Quality stated:

> The indoor organic air pollutants as reported from several large surveys are similar in the distribution of concentrations in residential environments in several industrialized countries."[31]

The Committee identified 73 chemicals commonly found in indoor air worldwide. Their complex names—hexane, formaldehyde, benzene, trichloroethylene, 1,1,1-trichloroethane, methyl ethyl ketone—can easily frighten people who believe themselves victimized, as well as company officials who are ultimately responsible for conditions in a building. However, these chemicals are seldom present in concentrations high enough to cause health problems.

Chamber studies have shown that air containing organic chemicals can cause eye and throat irritation.[32,33] However, the concentrations at which these occur are relatively high compared with levels detected in most indoor air—a fact also noted by the WHO report. Indoor air concentrations of substances are often thousands of times lower than those known to produce health effects. Occupational Safety and Health Administration (OSHA) regulations frequently permit industrial workers to be exposed to levels of chemicals hundreds or even thousands of times greater than the levels commonly detected in buildings; yet no adverse health effects are expected for the workers. When chemical concentrations are measured in buildings where the workers are complaining, the detected levels are often no higher than customary background levels measured in homes, shopping malls, and neighborhood restaurants.

If inadequate ventilation were responsible for reported symptoms, you would expect that increasing ventilation could solve or at least improve the situation. Researchers at the University of Toronto tested the relationship between reported symptoms and the amount of ventilation in four office buildings over a six-week period. Each week, the participants, unaware of the experimental intervention, reported symptoms and the indoor environment was thoroughly evaluated. The researchers found that increases in the supply of outdoor air did not appear to affect workers' perceptions of their office environment or their reporting of symptoms considered typical of SBS.[34]

Scientists who believe that indoor air problems pose a significant health threat have used flawed survey techniques to support that belief.

In a sample of workers conducted by Honeywell Technalysis, 24 percent of 600 workers perceived air quality problems in their offices.[35] Nearly 10 percent perceived the problems to be very serious, and 20 percent thought they impaired their productivity. Extrapolating these numbers, Dr. James Woods, an engineer at Virginia Tech University, suggests that 800,000 to 1,200,000 commercial buildings in the United States have problems that can cause "sick building syndrome" among 30 to 70 million exposed occupants.[36]

The problem with Woods's conclusion is that no cause-and-effect relationship has been established. Woods based his extrapolations and extensive recommendations on the assumption that an indoor air problem was responsible for the workers' symptoms. It is just as likely that emotional factors and reporting biases (increased awareness leading to increased complaints) were responsible. Yet this study has been widely quoted and has been accepted by medical and engineering professionals and by federal and state agencies that deal with environmental issues.

Too Many Cooks

Much confusion has resulted from the diversity of professionals involved in the relatively new area of indoor air quality. Indoor air issues are addressed by so many disciplines—medicine, toxicology, public health, industrial hygiene, engineering, and architecture—that expertise is diluted. Each field has its own interpretations and unique solutions. The result: no one oversees the big picture—a perfect scenario for expensive piecemeal solutions.

It is far easier to collect data than it is to interpret or act upon that data. Environmental engineering firms may be ill-equipped to interpret the potential public health effects of their findings. They are even less likely to be able to judge the significance of individual complaints. Because they are not health professionals, they cannot respond effectively to the concerns of the workers. As a result, the employer or building manager who retained them can be left with a set of data with no meaning and no rational basis for an action plan.

The number of indoor-air consultants is now in the thousands and is growing exponentially. Some are well-qualified and have a broad understanding of the relationship between health and environment.

Most, unfortunately, do not. They are quick to confirm health problems that do not exist and ready to consider whatever they uncover as the cause of those problems. This is often followed by expensive measures that bear no true relationship to the actual problem. Although hundreds of buildings have been evaluated, few investigations have led to clear-cut conclusions that could be used to implement effective corrective action.[3,37,38] Nevertheless, allegations of SBS have disrupted office staffs, undermined worker productivity, spawned a multimillion-dollar indoor-air assessment industry, and spearheaded calls for hundreds of millions of dollars for modifying buildings.

The Media's Role

The media coverage of building-related health issues reflects the general confusion surrounding the matter. They may mix deaths, asbestos, illnesses, and symptoms in a single story, leaving the impression that they are somehow all linked by a common disorder of indoor air. Most commonly, stories about indoor air are covered by local papers in response to complaints by workers or families of students. Frequently there is little scientific input in the story, often because the "problem" is unidentifiable. This may suggest that there is a mysterious and silent threat so pernicious that it defies detection. For example:

> *Environment: Your Office May be Hazardous*
> More and more Americans are becoming aware of air-quality hazards in the workplace, and terms such as "sick building syndrome" and "Legionnaires' disease" have entered the vernacular. But air pollution is only one threat among the many in the modern office. Recent research has revealed numerous other environmental factors with direct and indirect effects on human health and performance.
>
> *The Washington Post*
> September 17, 1989

> *Sick Building Syndrome: A Growing Risk to Workers*
> Jennifer, who sells specialized services for a New England-based computer manufacturer, used to be an active young adult before she moved into her new company's office complex more than a year ago.
>
> *San Francisco Chronicle*
> November, 23, 1990

Employee Group Seeks Cure for 'Sick' County Courthouse
The deaths of several courthouse workers and judges, and the mysterious illnesses that have plagued other employees, have sent Superior Court Clerk Church Martin looking for an antidote to the "sick building syndrome."
The Los Angeles Times
January 14, 1991

Although today's office environment is light years ahead of the office of the past, it has introduced its own unique dilemmas. Thirty to 50 years ago, the biggest work-related problems occurred when someone got injured operating machinery on the job. Today's office poses more insidious, less detectable threats — sick building syndrome; neck, back and wrist injuries; stress-related illnesses, and chronic fatigue syndrome.
The Buffalo News
July 1, 1997

Of course, the more attention the media give to this issue, the greater the number of workers who make complaints.

The Link to MCS

When people employed in a commercial or public building become ill, most soon recover regardless of the cause. For a few workers, however, the brush with an indoor environmental hazard—real or perceived—begins a downward spiral of persistent symptoms and a dysfunctional lifestyle. A significant fraction of the MCS population began their ordeal with a building-related problem.

The symptoms of SBS often resemble those of MCS. When studies fail to detect a level of chemicals or microorganisms that exceeds an established threshold for disease, the MCS diagnosis enables them to claim that they are more sensitive than the general population and therefore vulnerable to much lower levels.

References

1. Fraser DW and others. Legionnaire's disease: Description of an epidemic of pneumonia. New England Journal of Medicine 297:1189, 1977.
2. McDale JE and others. Legionnaire's disease: Isolation of a bacterium and demonstration of its role in other respiratory diseases. New England Journal of Medicine 297:1197, 1977.

3. Gots RE and others. Proving causes of illness in environmental toxicology: "Sick buildings" as an example. Fresenius Environmental Bulletin 1:135–142, 1992.

4. Ryan CM, Morro LA. Dysfunctional buildings or dysfunctional people: An examination of the sick building and allied disorders. Journal of Consulting & Clinical Psychology 60:220–224, 1992.

5. Rothman AL, Weintraub MI. The sick building syndrome and mass hysteria. Malingering and Conversion Reactions 13:405–412, 1995.

6. Brundage JF and others. Building-associated risk of febrile acute respiratory diseases in army trainees. JAMA 259:2108–2112, 1988.

7. Levy F. The medical approach to patients with IAQ problems. In Indoor Air '90: The Fifth International Conference on Indoor Air Quality and Climate, Toronto, July 29–Aug. 3, 1990, Vol. 5, pp. 327–331.

8. Gots RE. Toxic Risks: Science, Regulation and Perception. Boca Raton, Fla.: Lewis Publishers, 1992.

9. Mikatavage MA and others. Beyond air quality—Factors that affect prevalence estimates of sick building syndromes. American Industrial Hygiene Association Journal 56:1141–1146, 1995.

10. Hodgson MJ and others. Symptoms and microenvironmental measures in nonproblem buildings. Journal of Occupational Medicine 33:527–533, 1991.

11. Palonen J, Seppanen O. Design criteria for central ventilation and air-conditioning system of offices in cold climate. In Indoor Air '90: The Fifth International Conference on Indoor Air Quality and Climate, Toronto, July 29–Aug. 3, 1990, Vol. 4, pp. 299–304.

12. Nagda NL, Koontz MD, and Albrecht RJ. Effect of ventilation rate in a healthy building. IAQ '91, Healthy Buildings, Washington, D.C., Sept. 1991:101–107.

13. Baldwin ME, Farant JP. Study of selected volatile organic compounds in office buildings at different stages of occupancy. In Indoor Air '90: The Fifth International Conference on Indoor Air Quality and Climate, Toronto, July 29–Aug. 3, 1990, Vol. 2, pp. 665–670.

14. Farant JP and others. Environmental conditions in a recently constructed office building before and after the implementation of energy conservation measures. Applied Occupational Environmental Hygiene 7:93–100, 1992.

15. Collett CW, Ventresca JA, Turner S. The impact of increased ventilation on indoor air quality. IAQ '91: Healthy Buildings, Washington, D.C., Sept. 4–8, 1991:97–100.

16. Menzies RI and others. Sick building syndrome: The effect of changes in ventilation rates on symptom prevalence: The evaluation of a double blind experimental approach. In Indoor Air '90: The Fifth International Conference on Indoor Air Quality and Climate, Toronto, July 29–Aug. 3, 1990, Vol. 1, pp. 519–524.

17. Hodgson, MJ. The sick building syndrome. In Seltzer JM, editor. Occupational Medicine: State of the Art Reviews: Effects of the Indoor Environment on Health. Philadelphia: Henley & Belfus 10:177–194, 1995.

18. Chang C and others. The sick building syndrome. I. Definition and epidemiological considerations. Journal of Asthma 30:285–295, 1993.
19. Zhu K. "Sick building syndrome": An inappropriate term. Journal of Occupational Medicine 35:752, 1993.
20. Colligan MJ. The psychological effects of indoor air pollution. Bulletin of the New York Academy of Medicine 57:1014–1026, 1981.
21. Gots RE. Multiple chemical sensitivities: Distinguishing between psychogenic and toxicodynamic. Regulatory Toxicology & Pharmacology 24:S8–S15, 1996.
22. Finnegan MJ and others. The sick building syndrome: Prevalence studies. British Medical Journal 289:1573–1575, 1984.
23. Hedge A, Erickson WA. Predicting sick building syndrome at the individual and aggregate levels. Environment International 22:3–19, 1996.
24. Arnetz BB and others. Mental strain and physical symptoms among employees in modern offices. Archives of Environmental Health 52:63–67, 1997.
25. Corn M and others. Personal communication to Dr. Gots, 1991.
26. Nelson NA and others. Health symptoms and the work environment in four nonproblem United States office buildings. Scandinavian Journal of Work Environment and Health 21:51–59, 1995.
27. Lees-Haley PR. When sick building complaints arise. Occupational Health and Safety 62:51–54, 1993.
28. Wiliams CW, Lees-Haley PR. Perceived toxic exposure: A review of four cognitive influences on perception of illness. Journal of Social Behavior and Personality 8:489–506, 1993.
29. Pennybaker JW, Skelton J. Selective monitoring of bodily sensations. Journal of Personality and Social Psychology 41:213–223, 1981.
30. Pennybaker JW, Watson D. Self-reports and physiological measures in the workplace. In Hurrell JJ and others, editors. Occupational Stress: Issues and Developments in Research. New York: Taylor and Francis Publishers, 1988:184–199.
31. World Health Organization. Indoor Air Quality: Organic Pollutants. Report on a WHO Meeting, Berlin. Regional Office for Europe, Copenhagen. 1989.
32. Molhave L and others. Human reactions to low concentrations of volatile organic compounds. Environment International 12:167–175, 1986.
33. Molhave L. Controlled experiments for studies of the sick building syndrome. Annals of the New York Academy of Sciences 641:46–55, April 30, 1992.
34. Menzies RI and others. The effect of varying levels of outdoor-air supply on the symptoms of sick building syndrome. New England Journal of Medicine 328:821–827, 1993.
35. Woods JE and others. Office worker perceptions of indoor air quality effects on discomfort and performance. In Indoor Air '87: Proceedings of the Fourth International Conference on Indoor Air Quality and Climate, Berlin, Aug. 17–21, 1987, Vol. 2, pp. 464–468.

36. Woods JE. Cost avoidance and productivity in owning and operating buildings. In Cone JE, Hodgson MJ, editors. Problem Buildings: Building-Associated Illness and Sick Building Syndrome. Occupational Medicine State of the Art Review 4:575–592, 1989.
37. Stolwijk JAJ. The sick building syndrome. Department of Epidemiology and Public Health, Yale University School of Medicine. Unpublished report, 1990.
38. National Institute for Occupational Safety and Health (NIOSH). Indoor air quality and work environment study. Public Health Service, Centers for Disease Control and Prevention, HETA 88-364-2105, 1991.

7

Are America's
Children at Risk?

Not long ago, two children, ages eight and ten, living in Georgia, developed upper respiratory infections, the sort that all children get. Shortly before that, their mother had seen a television exposé which stated that indoor air pollution was a serious problem in schools. Instead of assuming that her children had been infected by run-of-the-mill viruses, she decided they were the victims of a toxic school. Since the television program had warned that most physicians were not attuned to these hazards, she bypassed her usual pediatrician and consulted a "special expert" in "environmental illness." The result was predictable. That physician diagnosed both children as "chemically sensitive" and advised the mother to make the following demands:

The children could not attend art classes.
They could only use special crayons.
There could be no pesticides used in the school.
No standard cleaning solutions could be used.
They could not ride on the school bus.
All carpeting had to be removed.

Continued questioning by the mother generated a growing list of symptoms, which led her to make further demands. The school administration granted some of them but refused others it considered unreasonable. Meanwhile, the children became increasingly isolated and were viewed by their classmates as "different." Eventually, an impasse developed and the mother filed a lawsuit stating that her children were ill and were entitled to special accommodation under state laws intended to help the handicapped. When the court disagreed, she withdrew the children from school and tutored them herself at home.

The MCS Connection

Concerns about "uniquely sensitive" children have injected the MCS movement into school systems nationwide. The typical elements are a routine illness, a worried parent caught up in a health scare, a supportive physician, and, frequently, an MCS support network. The children are often caught in the middle of a nasty confrontation and labeled—without foundation—as "abnormal," "different," or "disabled."

During the past several years, Dr. Ronald Gots has evaluated the cases of over a dozen children who were alleged to have "chemical sensitivity." Half of the evaluations were confined to reviewing medical records, and half also included examination of the child. All involved situations in which a court had been asked to decide whether these students had special needs that justified expensive and ever-escalating parental demands. In each case, it was claimed that the children were sensitive to pesticides, cleaning materials, and/or mold in their school. The suits were based on laws designed to protect the rights and accommodate the special needs of handicapped or disabled students. Gots found no evidence of physical disease related to anything in the schools. A few of the children had asthma, as do many children, but the allergens that prompted attacks were the pets and the dust in their homes.

Sometimes the lack of a connection is obvious to all but the participants. Gots's cases included two brothers, ages eleven and fifteen, whose mother thought they were being poisoned by chemicals in their schools and in the school buses. The school was sending a driver to pick up one of the boys because of his alleged sensitivity to exhaust fumes produced by the buses. However, the mother was suing for further accommodations. Both boys had a passionate interest in building cars—not models, but actual race cars that they drove around a track at up to 70 miles per hour. When asked about the fumes associated with this activity (weekly during the school year but more frequent during the summer), the boys replied—with apparent sincerity—that the wind always blew the car exhaust away from them.

The Healthy School Handbook

Perhaps the most dangerous expression of the notion of sick schools and victimized children is *The Healthy School Handbook*,[1] a 456-page work filled with unsubstantiated advice. The book was published by the National Education Association, a reputable professional organization that should have known better. It is an outgrowth of the 1992 annual meeting of the American Academy of Environmental Medicine, which devoted an entire day to sessions on "Environmental causes of learning, behavioral, and other health problems in school children." Published in 1995, it has become a manifesto for chemical sensitivity activists, a source of worry for countless parents, and a thorn in the side of school administrators.

The book was developed and edited by Norma Miller, Ed.D., a former art teacher whom the book described as an "education and environmental consultant" in Fort Worth, Texas. In the preface, Miller describes how exposure to perfume, hair-spray odors, sawdust, floor wax, mimeograph ink, art supplies, and cigarette smoke caused her to become so sensitive to chemical fumes that she resigned her teaching job. After partially recovering, she obtained a doctoral degree based on her research on "the top ten areas of concern associated with the construction and maintenance in healthful school buildings." In Chapter 4, which lists these concerns, she warns:

> Schools should not be built near major highways, railroads, airports, television or radio stations, microwave towers, high power electrical lines, toxic dumps, or garbage incinerators.[2]

Chapter 11 claims that exposure to electromagnetic fields (EMFs) increases the risk of developing cancer and that "some persons, particularly the old and the young, may be particularly susceptible." Claims of this type, however, are based on either flawed studies or pure guesswork. The chapter also states:

> The health risks due to EMFs go far beyond their role in causing cancer. They extend to other diseases, and also have a role in causing various symptoms that do not fit easily into specific diagnostic categories. It is probably the case that EMFs combine with other noxious stimuli and risk factors, thereby taxing the body's overall resistance to disease.[3]

An accompanying illustration shows a balloonlike structure bursting at the top when the "total load" of EMFs, radon, genes, asbestos, poor diet, and anger exceed the "body's adaptive capacity." This notion is nonsensical. The chapter's author recommends that classrooms be audited by "competent and independent engineers" to identify sources that can be removed. He also recommends using building materials that shield against EMFs from the outside and special shields that block EMF emission from computers. He fails to mention the many studies that led the National Radiological Protection Board to conclude that "the epidemiological data do not provide a basis for restricting human exposure to electromagnetic fields.[4,5]

The handbook contains many anecdotes about children who allegedly became disruptive following exposure to new carpets, the particle board of a computer table, perfume worn by teachers, and many other common items. The most vivid of these is the story of ten-year-old "Jared." According to the chapter's author:

> Jared . . . has been forced into the sheltered world of home-instruction because of a sensitivity to chemicals.
>
> This sensitivity causes Jared to act irrationally both at home and in the classroom. His disruptive behavior is characterized by periods of depression interspersed with aggressiveness. . . . His performance on his classwork is poor, his handwriting resembles scrawled pictures, and, at best, his attention span is limited to a few minutes. . . .
>
> Jared's problem results from exposure to an unidentified toxic chemical during his development in the womb, and both his doctor and his parents believe that a "bug bomb" used to kill cockroaches may have been the culprit. . . .
>
> Although the pesticide issue that affects Jared may sound far-fetched, it has serious impact on many students across America. Because a classroom is treated with "bug-spray," students exposed to toxins in the pesticide may be in jeopardy of losing a lifetime of normal activity.[6]

In Chapter 22, Mary Lamielle, who operates the National Center for Environmental Health Strategies (an MCS clearinghouse), advises anyone concerned about school pollution to become an "indoor air detective." She states:

> While faculty members and students are the most likely choices for this role, students at all grade levels should be taught to recognize problematic products and practices that might con-

taminate the indoor air, and to call for procedures and policies that are friendly to a healthier school building. . . .

Ideally, our "experts" might come together as part of an Indoor Air Quality Task Force or an Indoor Air Quality Team with the approval of the school administration. . . . This group should be charged with review of all products, practices, procedures, and policies that may affect a school's air quality.[7]

Lamielle's candidates for restriction include painting; roofing; floor-covering installation; all materials used for construction and remodeling; pesticides used in or near a school; fragranced or petrolatum-based cleaning products; solvent-based markers (used for drawing); freshly copied paper; Wite-Out® correction fluid; rubber cement; model glue; and personal products such as perfume, shampoo, hair spray, and clothing washed with a detergent or fabric softener.

The Feingold Connection

In 1973, Benjamin F. Feingold, M.D., a pediatric allergist from California, proposed that salicylates, artificial colors (especially tartrazine— Yellow #5), and artificial flavors caused hyperactivity in children. (Hyperactivity is now medically classified as attention deficit disorder [ADD] or attention deficit hyperactivity disorder [ADHD].) To treat or prevent this condition, Feingold suggested a diet that was free of such chemicals. In 1975, he popularized his theories with a book called *Why Your Child Is Hyperactive.*[8]

Feingold's ideas were based on personal observation rather than on clinical research. But as subsequently noted by allergist John C. Selner, M.D., and psychologist Herman Staudenmayer:

The tendency of non-critical minds (professional and lay) to universalize a clinical observation to a large subset of America's children achieved extraordinary momentum. Congressional committees were pressured by lay-interest groups, and the media began to give wide coverage to the reported connection between the ingestion of food and hyperactive behavior. Articles appeared in popular magazines, for example, the *Reader's Digest* Jekyll-and-Hyde cover story in the March 1981 issue. Even the prestigious *Wall Street Journal* gave page-one coverage to the matter on June 2, 1977. Feingold had touched a raw nerve that reached from the nation's boardrooms to its kitchens.[9]

ADDITIVES (800) 321-3287
can trigger
ADD (Attention Deficit Disorder)

FAUS bumper sticker.

Feingold's followers—many of whom belong to support groups—now claim that asthma, bedwetting, ear infections, eye-muscle disorders, seizures, sleep disorders, stomach aches, and a long list of other conditions may respond to the Feingold program and that sensitivity to synthetic additives and/or salicylates may be a factor in antisocial traits, compulsive aggression, self-mutilation, difficulty in reasoning, stuttering, and exceptional clumsiness. The table on the opposite page shows the symptoms listed as diet-related on the Feingold Association of the United States (FAUS) Web site in November 1997. The site also contains a long list of environmental chemicals to which it suggests children might be sensitive.

Adherence to the Feingold diet requires a change in family lifestyle and eating patterns, particularly for families who prepare many meals from "scratch." Feingold strongly recommended that the hyperactive child help prepare the special foods and encouraged the entire family to participate in the dietary program. Parents are also advised to avoid certain over-the-counter and prescription drugs and to limit their purchases of mouthwash, toothpaste, cough drops, perfume, and various other nonfood products to those published in FAUS's annual "Food List and Shopping Guide."

Current recommendations advise a two-stage plan that begins by eliminating artificial colors and flavors; the antioxidants BHA, BHT, and TBHQ; aspirin-containing products; and foods containing natural salicylates. If improvement occurs for four to six weeks, certain foods can be "carefully reintroduced" one at a time.[10] However, the *Feingold Cookbook* (published in 1979 but still in print) warns:

> A successful response to the diet depends on 100 percent compliance. The slightest infraction can lead to failure: a single bite or drink can cause an undesirable response that may persist for seventy-two hours or more.[11]

Many parents who have followed Feingold's recommendations have reported improvement in their children's behavior. FAUS, which has local chapters throughout the country, claims that fidgetiness, poor sleeping habits, short attention span, self-mutilation, antisocial traits, muscle incoordination, memory deficits, asthma, bedwetting, headaches, hives, seizures, and many other problems may respond to the Feingold program.[12] Despite these claims, carefully designed

Feingold Association Checklist for "Chemical Sensitivity"

The following symptoms are not to be considered abnormal—many people exhibit some of them at times. However, a truly chemically sensitive person will display more of them more frequently and to more of an extreme than the average person.

HYPERACTIVITY
Constant motion
Spinning or running in circles
Runs, does not walk
Difficulty sitting through meals
Wiggles legs/hands inappropriately

COMPULSIVE AGGRESSION
Disruptive at home & school
Doesn't respond to discipline
Doesn't recognize danger
Compulsively repeats action
Unkind to pets
Fights with other children
Poor self-control

POOR SLEEP HABITS
Difficult to get to bed
Hard to fall asleep; restless sleeper
Has nightmares, bad dreams

FREQUENT PHYSICAL COMPLAINTS
Headaches
Hives or rashes
Stomach aches
Ear infections
Bed wetting
Daytime wetting
Constipation/diarrhea

EMOTIONAL COMPLAINTS
Withdrawn
Miserable/depressed
Anxious/afraid

NEURO-MUSCULAR INVOLVEMENT
Accident-prone
Poor muscle coordination
Poor eye-hand coordination
Difficulty writing and drawing
Dyslexia
General learning disabilities
Difficulty with playground activities
Tics, twitches
Some forms of seizures
Walking on toes

IMPATIENCE
Low frustration tolerance
Demands must be met immediately
Irritable
Cries easily or often
Throws, breaks things

SHORT ATTENTION SPAN
Easily distracted
Doesn't finish projects
Doesn't listen to whole story
Doesn't follow directions

OTHER BEHAVIOR PROBLEMS
Unpredictable behavior
Impulsivity
Makes inappropriate noises
Talks too much
Talks too loudly
Interrupts
Overreacts to touch, pain, sound, lights
Jumping up and down (a lot)

experiments fail to support the idea that additives are responsible for such symptoms in the vast majority of children. Most improvement, if any occurs, appears related to changes in family dynamics, such as paying more attention to the children. Experts have also noted that the foods recommended in Feingold's 1975 book *Why Your Child Is Hyperactive* included some that were high in salicylates and excluded others that were low in salicylates.

In the ideal experiment, children whose behavior seems to have improved on the Feingold diet are kept on the diet but are periodically challenged with one or more suspected substances. Under ideal circumstances, the procedure should be double-blind, so that neither the participants nor the experimenters know when the substances are being administered. In 1980, an expert review team assembled by the Nutrition Foundation concluded:

> Based on seven studies involving approximately 190 children, there have been no instances of consistent, dramatic deterioration in behavior in hyperactive children challenged, under double-blind conditions, with artificial food colorings. . . . There are three . . . exceptions to these generally negative conclusions, but, in all three cases, the deterioration is reported by the mother with no other objective, confirming evidence available. . . . Without the confirming evidence of objective tests and/or outside observers, even these exceptions cannot be considered as definite evidence that there may be an occasional, genetically determined, sensitivity to food colorings. Though one cannot prove that no such children will be found, sufficient numbers of highly selected children have been studied to feel confident that such specific sensitivity, if found, will be rare.
>
> These negative findings stand in sharp contrast to the 32–60 percent of children reported by Dr. Feingold and others to improve dramatically under non-blind conditions without the use of placebo controls.[13]

In 1983, the review team's co-chairman and another colleague reviewed additional studies and concluded that no more than 2 percent of children respond adversely to food-color additives, and even that statistic was questionable.[14] Since that time, experimental findings have been mixed. Some researchers have reported no effect[15,16] and some have reported worsening behavior during challenge experiments.[17-19] However, it remains clear that the percentage of children who may become hyperactive in response to food additives is, at best, very small.

Sugar and aspartame (an artificial sweetener) have also been blamed for hyperactivity, but well-designed studies have found no evidence supporting such claims.[20-22]

The claims of Feingold advocates have steadily expanded, and some resemble those made by clinical ecologists. The *Feingold Handbook,* for example, states that "sensitivity to synthetic chemicals in the food or environment, or to some natural salicylates" can cause an adult to become a workaholic or to have nervous habits, chronic fatigue, impulsiveness, poor self-image, poor coordination, mental and physical sluggishness, temper flare-ups, headaches, depression, erratic sleep patterns, and a "tendency to interrupt."[12] These claims are absurd.

The September 1992 issue of the Feingold Association's newsletter, *Pure Facts*, claimed that teachers and children have been noted to suffer from the effects of chemicals used in construction, furnishing, housekeeping, maintenance, renovation, pest control, food service, and classroom activities at their schools. An article titled "The Sick Building Syndrome" stated that one child was repeatedly disciplined for reacting to his teacher's perfume, another child became abusive toward his mother because of the school's newly painted lunchroom, and that yet another child required tutoring because of a very bad reaction to a leak in the school's oil furnace. Although exposure to significant levels of chemical fumes in poorly ventilated buildings can make people ill, such instances are rare (see Chapter 6). The idea that perfume causes misbehavior is nonsensical.

Real Risks

Nobody wants children to be at risk in dangerous indoor environments. When threats are substantiated, or even strongly suspected (based on scientific evidence), protective measures are a logical response. On the other hand, unfounded fears can endanger the mental and physical well-being of children and can erode the fragile fiscal integrity of our school systems.

Children are directly victimized when scarce resources are allocated to managing phantom risks rather than improving programs, buying books, and buying computers. Others will be victimized if the cost of coping with unreasonable demands leads to tax increases.

Because the Feingold diet is physically harmless, it could be argued that there is nothing to lose by trying it. However, the potential benefits should be weighed against the potential harm of (1) teaching children that their behavior and school performance are related to what they eat rather than what they feel, (2) undermining their self-esteem by implanting notions that they are unhealthy and fragile, and (3) creating situations in which their eating behavior and fear of chemicals are regarded as peculiar by other children. Parental preoccupation with environmental factors can also prevent disturbed children from receiving appropriate professional help.

References

1. Miller NL, editor. The Healthy School Handbook: Conquering the Sick Building Syndrome and Other Environmental Hazards In and Around Your School. Washington, D.C.: National Education Association, 1995.
2. Miller N. Ten top concerns for a healthful school environment. In Miller NL, editor. The Healthy School Handbook: Conquering the Sick Building Syndrome and Other Environmental Hazards In and Around Your School. Washington, D.C.: National Education Association, 1995:63–80.
3. Marino AA. Electromagnetic fields in the classroom. In Miller NL, editor. The Healthy School Handbook: Conquering the Sick Building Syndrome and Other Environmental Hazards In and Around Your School. Washington, D.C.: National Education Association, 1995: 221–241.
4. National Radiological Protection Board. Electromagnetic fields and the risk of cancer. Summary of the views of the Advisory Group on Non-ionizing Radiation on epidemiological studies published since its 1992 report. NRPB 4(5):54, 1993.
5. Gandi OP, editor. Biological Effects and Medical Applications of Electromagnetic Energy. Englewood Cliffs, N.J.: Prentice Hall, 1990.
6. Forbes W. Jared's story: The least toxic approaches to managing pests in schools. In Miller NL, editor. The Healthy School Handbook: Conquering the Sick Building Syndrome and Other Environmental Hazards In and Around Your School. Washington, D.C.: National Education Association, 1995:243–254.
7. Lamielle M. Taking action: What you can do if your school building is sick. Miller NL, editor. The Healthy School Handbook: Conquering the Sick Building Syndrome and Other Environmental Hazards In and Around Your School. Washington, D.C.: National Education Association, 1995:409–421.
8. Feingold BF. Why Your Child Is Hyperactive. New York: Random House, 1975.

9. Selner JC, Staudenmayer H. The relationship of the environment and food to allergic and psychiatric illness. In Young SH and others, editors: Psychobiological Aspects of Allergic Disorders. New York: Praeger, 1986:102–146.

10. Food List and Shopping Guide: 1997. Alexandria, Va.: Feingold Association of the United States, 1996.

11. Feingold BF. The Feingold Cookbook for Hyperactive Children. New York: Random House, 1979.

12. The Feingold Handbook. Alexandria, Va.: The Feingold Association of the United States, 1986.

13. Wender EH, Lipton MA. The National Advisory Committee Report on Hyperkinesis and Food Additives—Final Report to the Nutrition Foundation. Washington, D.C.: The Nutrition Foundation, 1980.

14. Lipton MA, Mayo JP. Diet and hyperkinesis: A update. Journal of the American Dietetic Association 83:132–134, 1983.

15. Rowe KS. Synthetic food colourings and 'hyperactivity': A double-blind crossover study. Australian Paediatric Journal 24:143–147, 1988.

16. Gross MD and others. The effects of diets rich in and free from additives on the behavior of children with hyperkinetic and learning disorders. Journal of the American Academy of Child and Adolescent Psychiatry 26:53–55, 1987.

17. Carter CM and others. Effects of a few food diet in attention deficit disorder. Archives of Disease in Childhood 69:564–568, 1993.

18. Boris M, Mandel FS. Foods and additives are common causes of the attention deficit hyperactive disorder in children. Annals of Allergy 72:462–468, 1994.

19. Rowe KS, Rowe KJ. Synthetic food coloring and behavior: A dose response effect in a double-blind, placebo-controlled, repeated-measures study. Journal of Pediatrics 125:691–698, 1994.

20. Wolraich ML and others. Effects of diets high in sucrose or aspartame on the behavior and cognitive performance of children. New England Journal of Medicine 330:301–307, 1994.

21. Wolraich ML and others. The effect of sugar on behavior or cognition in children: A meta-analysis. JAMA 274:1617–1621, 1995.

22. Krummel DA and others. Hyperactivity: Is candy causal? Critical Reviews in Food Science and Nutrition 36(1–2):31–47, 1996.

8

The Mercury-Amalgam Scam

About half a century ago, Orson Welles panicked his radio audience by reporting that Martians had invaded New Jersey. On December 23, 1990, CBS-TV's "60 Minutes" achieved a similar effect by announcing that toxins had invaded the American mouth. There was, however, a big difference. Welles's broadcast was intended to be entertaining. The "60 Minutes" broadcast, narrated by veteran reporter Morley Safer, was intended to alarm—to persuade its audience that the mercury in dental fillings is poisonous. It was probably the most irresponsible report on a health topic ever broadcast on network television.

No Real Danger

Mercury is a component of the amalgam used for "silver" fillings. The other major ingredients are silver, tin, copper, and zinc. When mixed, these elements bond to form a strong, stable substance. Very sensitive instruments can detect billionths of a gram of mercury vapor in the mouth of a person with amalgam fillings. Although mercury—in certain forms and quantities—is a toxic substance, the minuscule amount the body absorbs from amalgams is far below the level that exerts any adverse health effect.[1,2]

The World Health Organization and the U.S. Occupational Safety and Health Administration (OSHA) have determined that the maximum "safe" dose is about 300 to 500 micrograms per day. People with a moderate to large number of fillings are exposed to 1 to 3 micrograms a

97

day, which is barely 1 percent of the dose considered safe. At this rate of decomposition, it would take about ten thousand years for the amalgams to dissolve completely.[3]

A recent study measured the exposure to mercury vapor among ten patients with symptoms attributed to their amalgam fillings and eight patients who had fillings but no reported health problems. The researchers measured the amount released over a thirteen-hour period and measured the mercury levels in the patients' blood plasma, red blood cells, and urine. The amount of mercury vapor absorbed was trivial, and the test results were similar in the two groups.[4] The potential exposure to mercury from dental amalgams is only about 10 percent of the normal daily intake from food, air, and water of a person who is not occupationally exposed.[5]

Since 1905, although billions of amalgam fillings have been used successfully, fewer than a hundred cases of localized allergic reactions have been reported in the scientific literature—and these usually subside within a few weeks. An extensive review published in 1993 by the U.S. Department of Health and Human services concluded that "there is scant evidence that the health of the vast majority of people with amalgam is compromised or that removing fillings has a beneficial effect on health."[6]

Dubious Claims

Despite these facts, a small but vocal group of dentists, physicians, and various other "holistic" advocates claim that mercury-amalgam fillings are a health hazard and should be replaced. The most outspoken advocate of such advice is Hal Huggins, D.D.S., of Colorado Springs, Colorado. Dr. Huggins graduated from the University of Nebraska School of Dentistry in 1962 and received a master of science degree from the University of Colorado in 1989.

Huggins has held many seminars for dentists on his notions about "balancing body chemistry" by nutritional methods. The basic premise of this approach is that many diseases and conditions can be prevented or cured by diet alone. In 1975, the American Dental Association Council on Dental Research concluded that there was little or no evidence to support Huggins's dietary claims.

In 1985, Huggins and his wife Sharon published a book, *It's All In Your Head*, which combines the discredited theories of balancing body

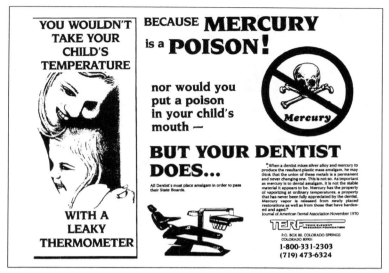

Flyer from Hal A. Huggins, D.D.S. The flyer is misleading because the mercury in fillings is chemically bound and is not released into the body in significant amounts.

chemistry with the assertion that mercury in silver fillings is toxic. The book states that he became interested in this subject in 1973 when a dentist from Argentina told him that leukemia, Hodgkin's disease, bowel disorders, and a host of other diseases had been cured by removing silver-mercury amalgams. Huggins says that early results were "sporadic and unpredictable. At best only 10 percent of the patients responded." Later he claimed that some fillings have "negative electrical current" and that removing fillings in the proper sequence and supplementing with nutrients would improve success rates. Since then he has crusaded against the use of amalgam and focused his practice on advice about this matter.

An information packet distributed during 1985 by Huggins's Toxic Element Research Foundation claims:

> Everyone reacts to the presence of mercury. . . . Some 80% of the population will experience only a slight change of their immune system which will result in three colds per winter instead of only two, or an elevation of 2000–3000 count in their white blood cells. Those sensitive 20% might experience a drastic drop in immunocompetence to the point of autoimmune disease, or an elevation of white blood cells of 30,000 or more.

According to Huggins, "sensitive" individuals can develop emotional problems (depression, anxiety, irritability), neurological disorders (facial twitches, muscle spasms, epilepsy, multiple sclerosis), cardiovascular problems (unexplained rapid heart rate, unidentified chest pains), collagen diseases (arthritis, scleroderma, lupus erythematosus), allergies, digestive problems (ulcers, regional ileitis), and immunologic disorders (which he claims include leukemia, Hodgkin's disease, and mononucleosis). He recommends replacing mercury fillings with other materials and taking vitamins and other supplements to prevent trouble following amalgam removal.

The Web site of Phillip P. Sukel, D.D.S., who practices in Arlington Heights, Illinois, lists about sixty "signs & symptoms of mercury vapor exposure from mercury amalgam dental fillings."[7] The list—like compilations for "multiple chemical sensitivity" and "candidiasis hypersensitivity"—includes abdominal cramps; allergies; anxiety; asthma; chronic or frequent headaches; cold, clammy hands and feet; colitis; decline of intellect; depression; diarrhea; dizziness; drowsiness; excessive perspiration; fatigue; irregular pulse; fine tremors; fits of anger; insomnia; irregular heart beat; irritability; nervousness; joint pain; lack of attention; loss of appetite; loss of weight; low self-confidence; low self-control; memory loss; muscle weakness; pain or pressure in chest; persistent cough; ringing in ears, shallow or irregular breathing; shyness/timidity; and sinusitis. There is no scientific evidence that mercury-amalgam fillings cause any of these problems.

Dubious Tests

Anti-amalgam dentists typically use a mercury vapor analyzer to convince patients that "detoxification," is needed. To use the device, the dentist asks the patient to chew vigorously for ten minutes, which may generate tiny amounts of mercury from the fillings. Although this exposure lasts for just a few seconds and most of the mercury will be exhaled rather than absorbed by the body, the machines give a falsely high readout, which the anti-amalgamists interpret as dangerous.

The most commonly used analyzer is an industrial device that multiplies the amount of mercury it detects in a small sample of air by a factor of 8,000. This gives a reading for a cubic meter, a volume far larger than the human mouth. The proper way to determine mercury exposure is to measure blood or urine levels, which indicate how much the body has absorbed and excreted. Scientific testing has shown that the amount of mercury absorbed from fillings is insignificant and that people with fillings excrete no more mercury than those without them. If mercury came out of amalgam fillings in the amounts claimed by the anti-amalgamists, the fillings would not be durable.

Some anti-amalgamists use a voltmeter to measure supposed differences in the electrical conductivity of the teeth. One such device—the "Amalgameter"—was sold by Huggins during the early 1980s. In 1985, after another company took over its marketing, the FDA concluded that the device was misbranded because accompanying literature alleged that it could be used to recommend the removal of dental fillings. In a regulatory letter, the agency said:

> There is no scientific basis for the removal of dental amalgams for the purpose of replacing them with other materials as described in your leaflet. . . . We consider your device as being directly associated with . . . a process that may have adverse health consequences when used for the purposes for which it was intended.

The FDA action may have crimped the marketing of the Amalgameter. However, it has had little effect on the misuse of such devices in dental offices.

Some anti-amalgamists have used mercury skin-patches to test for mercury "allergy" or "hypersensitivity." The patch contains a caustic chemical (mercuric chloride) that causes skin irritation, which the practitioner misinterprets as significant.

Dubious Ethics

In 1986, the American Dental Association Council on Ethics, Bylaws, and Judicial Affairs concluded that "removal of amalgam restorations for the alleged purpose of removing toxic substances from the body, when such treatment is performed at the recommendation of the dentist, presents a question of fraud or quackery in all but an exceedingly limited spectrum of cases." The ruling was triggered in part by the case of an Iowa dentist who had extracted all twenty-eight teeth of a patient with multiple sclerosis. The dentist received a nine-month license suspension followed by fifty-one months of probation.

Removing good fillings is not merely a waste of money. In some cases, it results in loss of teeth. In 1985, a $100,000 settlement was awarded to a fifty-five-year-old California woman whose dentist had removed her silver fillings. The dentist claimed that the fillings were a "liability" to her large intestine. In removing the fillings from five teeth, the dentist caused severe nerve damage necessitating root canal therapy for two teeth and extraction of two others.

Dubious Research

In 1990, researchers at the University of Calgary in Alberta, Canada, reported on an experiment in which they placed twelve amalgam fillings in each of six sheep. Within two months, the researchers claimed, the sheep lost much of their kidney function while a control group (two sheep) had lost none. *Newsweek*, which accepted the report at face value, described it as the first evidence that the amount of mercury escaping from fillings and winding up in body tissues is harmful. However, experts in biochemistry, toxicology, dentistry, and veterinary medicine consider the sheep study meaningless.

One of these authorities is Robert S. Baratz, D.D.S., Ph.D., M.D., an expert on dental materials. In a letter mailed to "60 Minutes" two weeks before its program was aired, he noted:

- The Canadian researchers prepared their amalgam with a method that has been obsolete for more than forty years. The resultant amalgam contained excess mercury and was softer and therefore more easily worn by chewing, especially in a cud-chewing animal such as a sheep.

- The amalgams were placed in opposing teeth, so they would grind against each other. This enhanced the already enhanced rate of release of materials.

- Because rubber dams were not used when the fillings were placed, scrap amalgam was free to enter the sheeps' mouth and be swallowed.

- The claim of kidney toxicity was based on urinary findings that show just the opposite of what is known to occur in mercury poisoning in humans.

• The methods used to detect and calculate the amount of mercury absorbed were not valid. Although the researchers claimed that body mercury levels rose during the experiment, they had not measured the levels that were present in the beginning. The data actually showed that the animals swallowed a lot of free mercury during the placement of the fillings.

Dr. Baratz and at least one other knowledgeable critic also spoke by telephone to producer Patti Hassler before the program was aired. But they encountered a stone wall.

Toxic Television

The "60 Minutes" segment on dental amalgam, which was considerably longer than most of its reports, was called "Poison in Your Mouth." It interspersed remarks from an American Dental Association representative with statements by three amalgam critics and four patients who claimed to have made a remarkable recovery from arthritis or multiple sclerosis after their amalgam fillings were removed. The most powerful segment featured a woman who said that her symptoms of multiple sclerosis had disappeared overnight. The fact that arthritis and multiple sclerosis normally have ups and downs was not mentioned during the program. Neither was the fact that removal of fillings temporarily raises body mercury load, so that no "overnight cure" could possibly be caused by mercury removal.

Not surprisingly, the broadcast triggered an avalanche of queries to dentists and induced many viewers to seek replacement of their fillings with other materials. *Consumer Reports, American Health, Prevention,* and several health newsletters reassured their readers that amalgam is safe. But the program's damage could not be undone. In August 1991, *Consumer Reports* published the following letter:

> My mother, who was diagnosed with Lou Gehrig's disease more than two years ago, had her mercury fillings removed immediately after the show aired. After she had spent $10,000 and endured more than 18 hours of dental work so painful she once fainted in the waiting room, her condition did not improve. The pain was outweighed only by the monumental disappointment she and the whole family experienced as we lived through one false hope.

In recent years, Hal Huggins has also targeted root canal therapy, claiming that it can make people susceptible to arthritis, multiple sclerosis, amyotrophic lateral sclerosis (Lou Gehrig's disease), and other autoimmune diseases. As with mercury-amalgam fillings, there is no objective evidence that teeth treated with root canal therapy have any adverse effect on the immune system or any other system or part of the body. Huggins's dental license was revoked in 1996. During the revocation proceedings the administrative law judge concluded: (1) Huggins had diagnosed "mercury toxicity" in all patients who consulted him in his office, even some without mercury fillings; (2) he had also recommended extraction of all teeth that had had root canal therapy; and (3) Huggins's treatments were "a sham, illusory and without scientific basis." Appendix G contains more information about the judge's ruling.

The Bottom Line

The false diagnosis of mercury-amalgam toxicity is potentially very harmful and reflects extremely poor judgment on the part of the practitioner. We believe that health professionals who engage in this practice should have their licenses revoked.

References

1. Mackert JR. Dental amalgam and mercury. Journal of the American Dental Association 122:54–61, 1991.
2. The mercury in your mouth. Consumer Reports 56:316–319, 1991.
3. Olsson S, Bergman M. Daily dose calculations from measurements of intra-oral mercury vapor. Journal of Dental Research 71:414–423, 1992.
4. Berglund A, Molin M. Mercury vapor release from dental amalgam in patients with symptoms allegedly caused by amalgam fillings. European Journal of Oral Science 104:56–63, 1996.
5. Mackert JR. Factors affecting estimation of dental amalgam exposure from measurements of mercury vapor in levels in intraoral and expired air. Journal of Dental Research 66:1175–1180, 1987.
6. Benson JS and others. Dental Amalgam: A Scientific Review and Recommended Public Health Strategy for Research, Education and Regulation. Washington, D.C.: U.S. Public Health Service, 1993.
7. Sukel PP. Phillip P. Sukel Online (http://www.sukel.com/mercury.htm), December 1997.

9

The Gulf War
Connection

Between August 1990 and June 1991, war in the Persian Gulf uprooted nearly 700,000 Americans and brought them into a hostile environment. Soon after returning, some began to experience debilitating illnesses. The most common symptoms were fatigue, muscle and joint pain, memory loss, and severe headaches. Congress responded by ordering the U.S. Department of Defense (DoD) and the Veterans Administration (VA) to set up registries to which Gulf War veterans could report on their health. In 1992, when several members of a reserve unit reported such symptoms, the Defense Department conducted an epidemiologic study and found no evidence of a specific disease outbreak. Nevertheless, more than 60,000 have registered with one or both agencies.[1]

Many of these veterans are said to be suffering from "Gulf War syndrome," an ill-defined condition that has enraged veterans' groups, inflamed the public and Congress, and spawned countless stories about mysterious ailments, heartless bureaucrats, and government conspiracies. The mass media's insatiable interest in such topics has nourished all sorts of speculations, and the Internet has enabled thousands of people to share their concerns. With nearly 700,000 potential victims plus another million or more family members and intimate friends, the issue remains politically heated. Some sufferers claim to have MCS. About 10,000 with undiagnosed health problems have applied for disability benefits.[2] About 10 percent of those who registered with the VA were not ill but merely chose to become part of the database.[3]

The Role of Coincidence

The Institute of Medicine of the National Academy of Sciences has concluded that the term "Gulf War syndrome" is inappropriate because it implies a singular disorder exclusive to Gulf War veterans.[4,5] Although no such disease pattern has been found, Gulf War service is being blamed for cancers, birth defects, multiple sclerosis, Lou Gehrig's disease, lupus erythematosus, depression, weight loss, weight gain, hair loss, graying hair, herpes, and more than a hundred other symptoms and conditions.

When health problems strike, it is human nature to search for explanations. The key question, of course, is whether these ailments were related to the war or would have occurred anyway. One way to investigate is to determine whether those who served in the war have a higher incidence of health problems than other troops or comparable civilians. In May 1995, President Bill Clinton established a twelve-person Presidential Advisory Committee on Gulf War Veterans' Illnesses composed of veterans, scientists, health-care professionals, and policy experts. By October 1996, approximately 62,000 individuals had completed physical examinations in the VA Persian Gulf Health Registry and the VA had reviewed the results for the first 52,216.[6] After examining these and other data, the committee concluded:

- Many veterans clearly are experiencing medical difficulties connected to their service in the Gulf War. Continuing to provide clinical care to evaluate and treat their service-connected illnesses is vital. However, a causal link between a single factor and the symptoms they report remains elusive.

- Veterans deployed to the Gulf reported more symptoms than did other veterans. However, no consistent laboratory or physical findings have been found in groups with increased symptoms. The most frequently reported symptoms were joint pain, fatigue, rash, headache, and memory loss, all of which are also common in the general adult population in the United States.

- Baseline data on military populations were not available, but it appears that the incidence of birth defects [normally about three percent of the general population] was not different among deployed and nondeployed groups.

- Objective tests of memory and concentration were the same or slightly lower among Gulf War groups, but self-perceptions of memory dysfunction were greater.

- After the war, Gulf War veterans had higher death rates from motor vehicle accidents and other external causes, but their death rates from all illnesses, including infectious diseases and cancer, have been the same or lower.[3]

The death-rate study upon which the above conclusion was based was published by the *New England Journal of Medicine* in March 1996.[7] An accompanying report concluded that during the two years after the war, the rate of hospitalization of Gulf War veterans remaining on duty did not differ significantly from that of other active-duty personnel.[8]

The Role of Stress

Some veterans—about ten thousand at last count—have symptoms that do not fit the patterns of specific diagnosable diseases. Yet that has happened after every major military conflict. In World War I, this symptom picture was called shell shock. In recent years, it has been called posttraumatic stress disorder (PTSD). Studies have shown that veterans deployed in the Gulf War have a higher rate of PTSD than either nondeployed veterans or the general U.S. population.

The key question is whether stress was a significant causal factor in many of the ill-defined Gulf War cases. The Presidential Advisory Committee concluded that it was. After earlier wars, the general public found such attribution acceptable, but today, emotional causes of disease carry a stigma. Thus a frantic search is under way for other explanations—many of them chemical. Researchers have been considering every conceivable risk factor: pesticides, chemical warfare agents, biological warfare agents, vaccines, pyridostigmine bromide (an anti-nerve gas agent), infectious diseases, depleted uranium, oil-well fires and smoke, petroleum products, psychologic and physiologic stress. More than a hundred federally funded studies and many privately funded studies of "Gulf War syndrome" have been launched, at a total cost of over $100 million. In December 1996, after reviewing all of the available data, the Presidential Advisory Committee concluded:

> Current scientific evidence does not support a causal link be-
> tween the symptoms and illnesses reported today by Gulf War
> veterans and exposures while in the Gulf region to the following
> environmental risk factors assessed by the committee: pesti-
> cides, chemical warfare agents, biological warfare agents, vac-
> cines, pyridostigmine bromide, infectious diseases, depleted
> uranium, oil-well fires and smoke, and petroleum products.
>
> Stress is known to affect the brain, immune system, cardio-
> vascular system and various hormonal responses. Stress mani-
> fests in diverse ways and is likely to be an important contributing
> factor to the broad range of physical and psychological illnesses
> currently being reported by Gulf War veterans.[3]

The committee also noted:

> Even when the war was over, many veterans experienced post-
> deployment stress on their return from the Gulf. These included
> financial and employment difficulties, unresolved military pay
> issues, the revelation of cases of leishmaniasis [a protozoal
> infection] and the consequent temporary ban on blood dona-
> tions, increasing numbers of health complaints and "unex-
> plained illnesses," and media accounts of apparent increased
> numbers of birth defects and cancer.

Thus the most comprehensive review to date concluded that stress
alone is the common link to the Gulf experience that could explain
symptoms. Furthermore, the committee's report indicts the media for
sensationalism and failure to accept the mounting scientific evidence. It
also viewed the media as a source of additional stress.

Elaine Showalter, distinguished professor of humanities at Princeton
University, classifies Gulf War syndrome with other "hysterical epidemics" including alien abductions, satanic ritual abuse, recovered memory,
and multiple personality syndrome.[9] Her book *Hystories: Hysterical
Epidemics and the Modern Media* includes the story of Gulf War veteran
Brian T. Martin, whose postwar symptoms have included excruciating
headaches; low back pain; diarrhea; burning and swelling of the feet;
blood in the stool; burning, swelling, and pain of the joints of the knees
and hands; mood swings; insomnia; getting lost when he drives; lumps
in the thigh, stomach, and rib cage; tinnitus (ringing in the ears);
debilitating fatigue; and vomiting in response to "perfumes, vapors,
other chemicals." Martin has also said he has been diagnosed with MCS,
sometimes forgets where he is, and needs a cane and wheelchair to get
around. Remarkably, Martin's wife has complained of rashes, headaches,

and unexplained symptoms she attributed to contact with her husband. She has supported this contention by stating that when her husband's semen touched her skin, "it would feel like it was on fire."[10]

Martin has been a major spokesperson for the Gulf War syndrome activists and a darling of the media. He has told his story on "Nightline," "60 Minutes," and Cable News Network, and in many newspaper and magazine interviews. Yet there have been clues that his story is implausible. The most important were disclosed at a 1996 Congressional hearing (see Appendix H), during which Martin said:

> It started in early 1991 with . . . blurred vision, shaking and trembling like I was on a caffeine high. My muscles were weakening, my chest pounded like my heart was going to explode through my chest. On Fort Bragg, during PT (physical training), I would vomit chem-lite looking fluids every time I ran, an ambulance would pick me up, putting IV's in both arms and rushing me to Womack Community Hospital. This happened EVERY morning after my return from the war.[11]

Chemlites are tubes containing chemicals that glow brightly for several hours when activated. In *Reason* magazine and the *Wall Street Journal*, investigative reporter Michael Fumento noted that, in two interviews, Martin had repeatedly described his vomit as "fluorescent."[12,13] In subsequent e-mail messages to Fumento, Martin denied using that word and said, "I was talking about color. Bile is almost the same color of certain Chemlites." (If so, we wonder why he didn't simply say "bright green.") He acknowledged, however, that the vomiting episodes had been "two to three times a week" rather than "EVERY" day.

Blurred vision, shaking, trembling, and pounding of the heart are typical of anxiety attacks (also called panic reactions), in which a sudden release of adrenaline (a hormone) into the bloodstream causes responses throughout the body. Although Martin probably has some physical problems as well, his countless symptoms do not constitute a syndrome, and most of them could not possibly result from exposure to an environmental toxin. Yet the media have portrayed him as typical of thousands of "forgotten" victims of an alleged government conspiracy.

In 1997, the *Journal of the American Medical Association* published three studies that have attracted considerable media attention. Funded by Ross Perot, the studies purportedly demonstrate relationships between certain neurological findings in a group of Gulf veterans and the use of pyridostigmine bromide and certain pesticides.[14-16] The studies had serious methodological problems that were criticized in a flurry of letters to the journal's editor.[17-19] Most of the patients had no findings according to the usual diagnostic methods, and there was little actual proof that they had been exposed to the alleged causal agents. Nevertheless, these reports and more that are likely to follow, have given new hope to veterans who would much prefer to have been poisoned than to be labeled as suffering from stress.

The MCS Connection

Ever vigilant for new recruits, MCS advocates have embraced "Gulf War syndrome" as their own. But the Presidential Advisory Committee on Gulf War Veterans' Illnesses has found no connection. In fact, its 174-page book dismisses MCS in two paragraphs:

> There is no consensus case definition for MCS, although two recent government-sponsored conferences have attempted to develop one. MCS patients report many symptoms, including tiredness, lethargy, fatigue, memory difficulties, difficulties concentrating, dizziness or lightheadedness, and depressed feelings when exposed to low levels of common, everyday substances. Symptoms relevant to many different organ systems have been linked to MCS in the clinical ecology literature; symptoms related to the central nervous system are the most common.
>   The majority of patients diagnosed with MCS have no objective abnormalities on physical examination or on routine laboratory testing. The physicians who use this diagnosis use a variety of nontraditional diagnostic and treatment techniques, none of which have been validated in a controlled trial.[3]

The Presidential Advisory Committee report has not settled the issue. Although the trail remains cold, conspiracy theories and claims that Gulf War syndrome is a strange or new disease (or is MCS) still flourish. Research projects are still under way, and President Clinton has announced that he will appoint another panel.[20]

In 1997, the Subcommittee on Human Resources of the House Government Reform and Oversight Committee complained that VA disability payments were being minimized by basing them on diagnoses of somatoform disorder and PTSD, which carry lower compensation ratings than those of physiologic ailments. This conclusion appears to have been influenced by the testimony of MCS advocates at hearings held by subcommittee chairman Christopher Shays (R-Conn.) during the past two years. On October 31, 1997, the subcommittee recommended passage of a law establishing a legal presumption that Gulf War veterans were exposed to chemicals and other hazardous substances—a law that would make it easier for them to collect disability benefits.[21] Commenting on this, Roy DeHart, M.D., past-president of the American College of Occupational and Environmental Medicine warned: "I don't know where you would draw the line. . . . Does a complaint equal a condition? For many people, that is all they have."[2]

The Bottom Line

The concept of a "Gulf War syndrome" is appealing. It comes at a time when public distrust of government is at an all-time high. It turns on conspiracies, a favorite theme of television producers. It provides the media with an endless parade of self-perceived victims. It provides a feeding trough for serious scientists, since funding is abundant, and for every charlatan with a newsworthy theory. It is a field day for politicians who solemnly promise to "get to the bottom" of the problem. The big losers in all of this are the ailing veterans whose confusion about what happened prevents them from getting on with their lives.

The same thing can be said about many people linked to the other fad diagnoses discussed in this book.

References

1. Congressional Research Service. Gulf War Veterans' Illnesses, 95–450 SPR, April 11, 1997:2.
2. Stapleton S. Panel to monitor Pentagon's handling of Gulf War illnesses. American Medical News 40(44):5–6, 1997.
3. Presidential Advisory Committee on Gulf War Veterans' Illnesses: Final Report. Washington, D.C.: U.S. Government Printing Office, Dec. 1996.
4. Institute of Medicine. Health Consequences of Service During the Persian Gulf War: Initial Findings and Recommendations for Immediate Action. Washington, D.C.: National Academy Press, 1995.
5. Institute of Medicine. Evaluation of the Department of Defense Persian Gulf Comprehensive Clinical Evaluation Program. Washington, D.C.: National Academy Press, 1996.

6. Kang HK and others. Health Surveillance of Persian Gulf War Veterans: A Review of the DVA Persian Gulf Registry Data. Unpublished report, Department of Veterans Affairs, March 1996.

7. Kang HK, Bullman TA. Mortality among U.S. veterans of the Persian Gulf War. New England Journal of Medicine 335:1498–1504, 1996.

8. Gray GC and others. The postwar hospitalization experience of U.S. veterans of the Persian Gulf War. New England Journal of Medicine 335(20):1505–1513, 1996.

9. Showalter E. Hystories: Hysterical Epidemics and Modern Culture. New York: Columbia University Press, 1997.

10. France D. The families who are dying for our country. Redbook, Sept. 1994:114–117, 147–148.

11. Martin BT. Prepared statement, Sept. 19, 1996. In The Status of Efforts to Identify Persian Gulf War Syndrome: Hearings before the Subcommittee on Human Resources and Intergovernmental Relations of the Committee on Government Reform and Oversight, House of Representatives, March 11, 28; June 25; and Sept. 19, 1996. Washington, D.C.: U.S. Government Printing Office, 1997:323–325.

12. Fumento M. Gulf Lore syndrome: Why are the Gulf War vets getting sick? You won't find out by reading the New York Times and USA Today. Reason, March, 1997.

13. Fumento M. Gulf War syndrome and the press. Wall Street Journal, March 4, 1997.

14. Haley RW and others. Is there a Gulf War syndrome? Searching for syndromes by factor analysis of symptoms. JAMA 277:215–222, 1997. Correction: JAMA 278:388, 1997.

15. Haley RW and others. Evaluation of neurologic function in Gulf War veterans: A blinded case-control study. JAMA 277:223–230, 1997.

16. Haley RW, Kurt TL. Self-reported exposure to neurotoxic chemical combinations in the Gulf War: A cross-sectional epidemiologic study. JAMA 277:231–237, 1997.

17. Hyams KG, Wignall FS. Identification of Gulf War syndrome: Methodological issues and medical illnesses. Letter to the editor. JAMA 278:384, 1997.

18. Amato AA, McVey A. Identification of Gulf War syndrome: Methodological issues and medical illnesses. Letter to the editor. JAMA 278:384, 1997.

19. Gots RE and others. Identification of Gulf War syndrome: Methodological issues and medical illnesses. Letter to the editor. JAMA 278:384, 1997.

20. Fumento M. A Sixth opinion: Unimpeded by science, a presidential panel will declare that Gulf War syndrome is real. Reason, Feb. 1998:46–47.

21. Shays C and others. Gulf War Veterans' Illnesses: VA, DOD Continue to Resist Strong Evidence Linking Toxic Causes to Chronic Health Effects. Washington, D.C.: House Government Reform and Oversight Committee, Nov. 7, 1997. Washington, D.C.: U.S. Government Printing Office, 1997.

Appendix A

A Double-Blind Study of Symptom Provocation to Determine Food Sensitivity

Abstract. *Background.* Some claim that food sensitivities can best be identified by intradermal injection of extracts of the suspected allergens to reproduce the associated symptoms. A different dose of an offending allergen is thought to "neutralize" the reaction.

Methods. To assess the validity of symptom provocation, we performed a double-blind study that was carried out in the offices of seven physicians who were proponents of this technique and experienced in its use. Eighteen patients were tested in 20 sessions (two patients were tested twice) by the same technician, using the same extracts (at the same dilutions with the same saline diluent) as those previously thought to provoke symptoms during unblinded testing. At each session three injections of extract and nine of diluent were given in random sequence. The symptoms evaluated included nasal stuffiness, dry mouth, nausea, fatigue, headache, and feelings of disorientation or depression. No patient had a history of asthma or anaphylaxis.

Results. The responses of the patients to the active and control injections were indistinguishable, as was the incidence of positive

---

From: Jewett DL and others. A double-blind study of symptom provocation to determine food sensitivity. New England Journal of Medicine 323:429–433, 1990.

responses: 27 percent of the active injections (16 of 60) were judged by the patients to be the active substance, as were 24 percent of the control injections (44 of 180). Neutralizing doses given by some of the physicians to treat the symptoms after a response were equally efficacious whether the injection was of the suspected allergen or saline. The rate of judging injections as active remained relatively constant within the experimental sessions, with no major change in the response rate due to neutralization or habituation.

Conclusions. When the provocation of symptoms to identify food sensitivities is evaluated under double-blind conditions, this type of testing, as well as the treatments based on "neutralizing" such reactions, appears to lack scientific validity. The frequency of positive responses to the injected extracts appears to be the result of suggestion and chance.

The diagnosis of food allergies and other sensitivities by provoking symptoms with injections of extracts of the suggested allergen[1-3] is a procedure so controversial[4] that its efficacy and theoretical basis have been reviewed by the California Medical Association[5] and the American Academy of Allergy.[6] Among the physicians using provocation testing or neutralization treatment are members of the American Academy of Environmental Medicine (formerly the Society for Clinical Ecology) and the Academy of Otolaryngic Allergy. Although a number of studies have been unable to confirm the validity and reproducibility of the symptom-provocation procedure,[7-9] these studies have been criticized by proponents[10,11] because the provocation techniques used did not duplicate those used in clinical practice (even though the technique as practiced differs from office to office). In response to this controversy, we designed and implemented a double-blind study that duplicated the procedures used in clinical practice. Before undertaking the study, we sent the protocol to both advocates and critics of provocation testing and modified it until most agreed that it was a fair and appropriate test of the method. That the protocol was acceptable to the proponents of provocation testing was evidenced by the participation of clinicians who used the method and by financial support from the Academy of Otolaryngic Allergy and the Society for Clinical Ecology.

Methods

Protocol. The protocol had four main features. First, it was carried out in the offices of seven experienced clinical ecologists in private practice who were proponents of symptom-provocation testing. Each had at least five years' experience with the technique. Second, only patients in whom symptoms had been consistently provoked during previous unblinded testing were studied. Patients were retested in the same office, by the same technician, who used the same extracts (at the same dilutions with the same diluent) as those found to provoke symptoms during unblinded clinical testing. Third, the study was double-blinded: The technician, the patients, and the investigator or observer had no knowledge of the contents of the syringes. Finally, each patient received a sufficient number of injections that the results for an individual patient could be analyzed for statistical significance without reference to the results in other patients, to permit the identification of a possible lone "responder."

Patients. All procedures were approved by the University of California, San Francisco, Committee on Human Research, and all patients gave informed consent. Eighteen patients were studied in seven private-practice offices throughout the United States. All patients were between 18 and 60 years of age, had no history of anaphylactic or anaphylactoid reactions, fainting, documented cardiac irregularity, severe laryngeal edema, severe asthma, or epileptic or epileptoid seizures; were recommended for the study by their physician on the basis of previous positive responses to intradermal or subcutaneous injections of "active" substances; and had had no symptoms in response to unblinded injections of the diluent alone. The 18 patients were studied 20 times (2 were studied twice, on different days). Fifteen of the patients were women and three were men.

On the day of the double-blind testing the physician had the option of conducting unblinded provocation testing earlier in the day and excluding the patient from the study if he or she did not respond as in previous clinical testing. None of the physicians chose to conduct such unblinded testing, and none withdrew any patient from the study, though the physicians could also have done so on the basis of a patient's self-reported condition on that day.

Procedures. The substances for the active injection, its concentration, and the method of the injection were chosen for each patient by his or her physician on the basis of the patient's previous unblinded clinical tests. These data are presented in Table 1. Of the 20 testing sessions, "underdoses" of the active substance were given in 17, and "overdoses" in 3. These doses were relative to a "neutralizing dose," defined as the dose that when injected in a volume of 0.1 ml, resulted in a wheal of 7 to 8 mm, which enlarged by 2 mm in 10 minutes. Thirteen patients were tested with foods, two with yeast, one with "mold A," and two with ethanol. The injections were given intradermally in 16 testing sessions and subcutaneously in the other 4. The diluent was normal saline, though whether it contained preservative or not depended on the routine practice at each office.

Although routine clinical skin testing normally takes three hours (usually with testing of five or six different substances), we wished to minimize the number of active injections and consequent discomfort. With an observation period of 10 minutes after each injection and several more minutes for recovery after symptom provocation, only four or five injections could be made in an hour. For a conservative limit of 12 injections, we chose to use a protocol with three active and nine control injections. With this protocol, the results for an individual patient could reach statistical significance (with Fisher's exact test) under the following circumstances: perfect identification of all active and placebo injections ($P < 0.0045$), one false positive and no false negative results ($P < 0.018$), two false positive and no false negative results ($P < 0.045$), and no false positive and one false negative result ($P < 0.045$).

One of the authors acted as an observer to ensure that the procedures were strictly adhered to; he also recorded the time course and occurrence of the patients' orally reported symptoms. For each test, a tray was prepared with 12 unmarked syringes. Each of the three syringes with active injections was assigned randomly (by a combined die-and-coin toss) to 1 of the 12 positions on the tray. The remaining syringes were filled with diluent. The technician who prepared the syringes placed the code in a sealed envelope, which was given to the observer but not opened until the testing was completed. This technician was the only one who knew the injection sequence. A different technician then used the syringes in order (1 through 12) and alternated the injections between arms; the first side injected was decided by the flip of a coin. The

Table 1. Responses of 18 Patients Forced to Decide Whether Injections Contained an Active Ingredient or Placebo.

| | | | | | NEUTRALIZING | | RESPONSES TO INJECTIONS | | | | |
| | | | | | DOSE | | ACTIVE | | PLACEBO | | P |
PT#	SEX	SUBSTANCE	ROUTE	DOSE	DOSE	OFFICE #	YES	NO	YES	NO	VALUE
3	F	Chocolate	ID	Under	Yes	2	2	1	1	8	0.13
1	F	Wheat	SC	Under	No	1	2	1	2	7	0.24
14a	F	Bakers' yeast	ID	Under	No	5	2	1	2	7	0.24
12	M	Potato	ID	Under	No	5	1	2	0	9	0.25
16	F	Ethanol	ID	Over	No	6	2	1	3	6	0.36
18	F	Ethanol	ID	Under	No	7	2	1	4	5	0.50
14b	F	Brewers' yeast	ID	Under	No	5	1	2	2	7	0.87
4	F	Chocolate	ID	Under	Yes	2	1	2	2	7	0.87
5	F	Wheat	ID	Under	Yes	2	1	2	2	7	0.87
9	F	Apple	ID	Under	No	2	0	3	0	9	
2a	M	Milk	SC	Under	No	1	0	3	1	8	0.75
13	M	Bakers' yeast	ID	Under	No	5	0	3	1	8	0.75
15	F	Wheat	ID	Under	No	6	1	2	3	6	0.76
6	F	Corn	ID	Under	Yes	2	0	3	2	7	0.55
8	F	Beef	ID	Under	Yes	2	0	3	2	7	0.55
17	F	Mold A	ID	Under	No	7	1	2	5	4	0.50
2b	M	Wheat	SC	Over	No	1	0	3	3	6	0.38
7	F	Orange	ID	Under	Yes	2	0	3	3	6	0.38
10	F	Potato	ID	Under	Yes	3	0	3	3	6	0.38
11	F	Chicken	SC	Over	No	4	0	3	3	6	0.38
Totals	—	—	—	—	—	—	16	44	44	136	0.78

PATIENT #: Patients were numbered in the order they were studied. The order in the table is related to the degree that the results agree with the hypothesis that patients could distinguish active injections from placebo injections. The results listed below those of patient 9 do not support this hypothesis: Placebo injections were identified as active at a higher rate than were true active injections. The letters "a" and "b" denote the first and second testing sessions, respectively, in patients 2 and 14.

ROUTE: ID denotes intradermal, and SC subcutaneous.

DOSE: An underdose was one that was lower than the neutralizing dose, and an overdose one that was higher.

NEUTRALIZING DOSE: Amount that, injected in a volume of 0.1 ml, resulted in a wheal of 7 to 8 mm and that enlarged by 2 mm in 10 minutes. Neutralizing doses were given to some patients after they reported symptoms.

P VALUE: Calculated according to Fisher's exact test, which assumes that the hypothesized direction of effect is the same as the direction of effect in the data. Therefore, when the effect is opposite to the hypothesis, as it is for the data below those of Patient 9, the P value computed is testing the null hypothesis that the results obtained were due to chance as compared with the possibility that the patients were more likely to judge a placebo injection as active than an active injection. The total P value is the P value associated with the test of whether the common odds ratio (the odds ratio for all patients) is equal to 1.0. The common odds ratio was equal to 1.13 (computed according to the Mantel-Haenszel test).

injections were separated by at least 10 minutes. After each injection, the injection site was covered, and the observer recorded any symptoms reported by the patient at one-minute intervals for 10 minutes. At the end of the 10-minute period the patient had to decide whether the injected substance had been active or control. The symptoms reported by the patients that were associated with an injection presumed to be active included itching of the nose, watering or burning eyes, plugged ears, a feeling of fullness in the ears or ringing ears, a dry mouth, a tight or scratchy throat, an odd taste in the mouth, tiredness, headache, nausea, dizziness, epigastric discomfort, scalp or facial tingling, a feeling of tightness or pressure in the head, disorientation, difficulty breathing, sleepiness, depression, chills, coughing, jaw tightening, nervousness, tension, intestinal gas or rumbling, and aching legs. If the patient reported that the substance was active (i.e., that symptoms had been provoked), then the next injection was delayed for 10 minutes. At the end of that time, the patient indicated whether the symptoms had cleared. If so, testing recommenced, if not, the injection was delayed for another 10 minutes. This process continued until the patient reported that the symptoms had subsided to baseline. Some physicians administered an unblinded, predetermined neutralizing dose to patients reporting symptoms. Neutralizing injections were given, after any injection (active or control) judged to be active, to seven patients in two offices (Table 1).

To analyze the data for all patients, we used the Mantel-Haenszel test to compute the common odds ratio.[12] The odds ratio—the odds of the patient's reporting symptoms after an active injection divided by the odds of the patient's reporting symptoms after a control injection—measures the size of the effect. Questions concerning habituation of responses and the effects of neutralization on subsequent injections were addressed by examining the odds of eliciting a symptom on the second and on the third active injection.

Results

Table 1 shows the patients' responses as well as the probability of obtaining such responses under the null hypothesis (no difference in the numbers of injections judged to be active or control). Across all sessions, the proportion of injections judged to be of the active substance was independent of the contents of the syringes. Twenty-seven percent of the active injections (16 of 60) were judged to be the active substance, as were 24 percent of the control injections (44 of 180). The strongest association in an individual patient (Patient 3) between reports of symptoms and active injections yielded a probability due to chance of 0.13 associated with an odds ratio of 9.4. One would expect results with this probability to occur by chance alone two to three times in 20 test sessions. Thus, none of our patients were unequivocal "responders" on the day of testing. The symptoms that were provoked were generally unrelated to the contents of the syringes. Furthermore, the overall results were quite random. One patient (Patient 9) reported no symptoms after any injection. Nine of the 20 sessions (45 percent) had a greater frequency per injection of reports of symptoms after active injections than after placebo injections (Patients 1, 3, 4, 5, 12, 14, 16, and 18) (Table 1), whereas another 9 sessions (45 percent) had exactly the opposite results (Patients 2, 6, 7, 8, 10, 11, 13, and 17) (Table 1). There were no consistent differences in results according to sex, substance injected, route of injection, or testing location (office), as can be determined from the results shown in Table 1. It is unlikely that the results were influenced by sensations at the injection site, since itching was reported at the site by only three patients (for 1 injection each), and stinging by nine patients (median, 3 injections; range, 1 to 12).

The Mantel-Haenszel test for homogeneity of the odds ratios was not significant ($P = 0.76$, $c^2 = 12$, $df = 16$), providing no evidence for an underlying distinction between "responders" and "nonresponders" in the study group. The results were consistent with the data having come from a single population in which the best estimate of the mean population (common) odds ratio is 1.13 (i.e., the odds of reporting symptoms after an active injection are 1.13 times the odds of reporting symptoms after a control injection). With this experimental paradigm, if the population odds ratio were 1.0 (i.e., no effect whatsoever), a sample overall odds ratio as divergent from 1.00 as 1.13 would occur more than 75 percent of the time ($c^2 = 0.03$, $df = 1$). Even if the sample odds ratio of 1.13 were the true population odds ratio, this would reflect a tiny effect. If this effect were present in the analysis of data from any individual patient, with three times as many control injections as active injections, one would need 726 active injections and 2,178 control injections to have an 80 percent probability of detecting this effect at the 0.05 level of statistical significance. Thus, an effect of this size could have no clinical usefulness.

Among the seven patients who were given neutralizing doses, the rate of false positive results was actually greater than the rate of true positive results. Most of the time, the neutralizing dose was given after symptoms had been "provoked" by a control (diluent) injection. The neutralizing dose was as effective in relieving these symptoms as it was in relieving those occurring after an active injection. In most cases a single neutralizing injection relieved the symptoms, and in no instance were more than two neutralizing doses administered. The injection of a neutralizing dose did not affect the sensitivity of the test procedure; the incidence of symptoms provoked after the neutralizing doses was similar to the overall rate and did not differ between active and control injections: 24 percent for active injections (4 of 17) and 23 percent for control injections (12 of 53).

The provocation of symptoms by either a control or an active injection did not significantly change the likelihood of patients' reporting symptoms after subsequent control or active injections. Thirty percent of the patients (6 of 20) accurately identified the first active injection, whereas 25 percent (5 of 20) accurately identified the first control injection. The accuracy of the identification of subsequent active injections was comparable: 30 percent (6 of 20) for the second active injection and 20 percent (4 of 20) for the third active injection. None of the differences was statistically significant. We thus conclude that the results did not reflect changes in sensitivity due to neutralization, habituation, or otherwise undefined "symptom fatigue."

Differences in the routes of injection—subcutaneous or intradermal—had no apparent effect on the rate of the occurrence of symptoms, though only a large effect could have been detected, since only three patients received subcutaneous injections. Similarly, there were no differences in the rate of occurrence of symptoms after an overdose or underdose of the active substance. Despite concern that an overdose might be detected by the patients, such injections were not associated with the occurrence of symptoms any more frequently than were control injections.

All seven of the participating offices were equally unsuccessful in providing a patient whose symptoms were reliably correlated with the syringe contents under double-blind conditions. We thus have no reason to suspect that differences in technique between offices somehow affected our results.

In looking for more subtle effects of the injections, we wondered whether the duration of symptoms provoked by active injections differed from that of control injections. Since the patients' symptoms were recorded minute by minute, we computed the number of minutes that symptoms persisted after the two types of injection. There was no significant difference in the duration of symptoms after active as compared with control injections. Reported symptoms lasted a mean (±SD) of 1.9 ± 2.1 minutes after active injections and 1.5 ± 1.3 minutes after control injections ($P > 0.15$). We did not observe any major differences in the magnitude of reported symptoms, but we did not study this systematically.

Discussion

Some have claimed that food allergies can best be identified by the so-called provocation-neutralization method, which "consists in the production of symptoms by giving an intracutaneous injection of a provoking dose of the food extract, then relieving these symptoms by giving successive intracutaneous injections of other dilutions of the same food extract, until the neutralizing dose is found."[13] The symptoms produced include headache, a feeling of nasal stuffiness, malaise, depression, fatigue, yawning, gas, discomfort, bloating, belching, feelings of anger, memory loss, a feeling of submissiveness, and tightness in the chest.[14] Kailin and Collier have reported that neutralizing injections relieved such symptoms more than 70 percent of the time; however, control (diluent) injections produced a similar rate of relief.[15] Our study was designed to duplicate the provocation-testing procedures used in clinical practice, as a further test of this method of diagnosis. We certainly did not expect the results that we obtained in these studies, since we had observed unblinded clinical testing in which active injections seemed to provoke symptoms readily. In our study, the active injections did provoke symptoms, but at a surprisingly low rate (27 percent), whereas the control (diluent) injections provoked symptoms at a surprisingly high rate (24 percent).

We had expected the rate of reaction to the diluent to be much lower, since previous testing was a requirement of entry into the study. However, the diluent injection had been tested without blinding only once or twice in each patient, and thus we have no good measure of the control reaction rate. We do not believe that the symptoms were provoked by something in the saline diluent, for the following reasons. First, only 25 to 30 percent of the injections provoked symptoms. Second, the patients did not respond to the diluent injection in the unblinded testing. Third, the patients' symptoms were relieved by the neutralizing dose, which contained a concentration of diluent identical to that of the provoking injection. If the biologic effects are related to the concentration of some hypothesized contaminant in the injections, then the concentration that provokes symptoms cannot be the same as the one that neutralizes them. Willoughby[16] has indicated that a dose that provokes symptoms can be considered to neutralize them as well, if the symptoms disappear within 20 minutes; however, he does not describe a single concentration that rapidly provokes and rapidly neutralizes symptoms. Finally, if all the bottles containing diluent contained a substance that would provoke symptoms, it is difficult to imagine a mechanism by which patients, in unblinded testing, could have been found to be sensitive to some "active" agents and not others (which have the same diluent). For these reasons, we conclude that the symptoms provoked by the control and active injections were unrelated to any substance present in all bottles. Rather, we propose a simpler explanation of the results: The symptoms were placebo responses, generated spontaneously. In one review of a number of studies involving a total of 1,082 subjects with conditions ranging from headache to postoperative wound pain, the placebo response rate was found to range from 15 to 58 percent, with an average (±SD) of 35±2 percent.[17]

Our study would have been even more powerful if all the patients had been studied on two days (with three active and nine control injections on each day): one day under unblinded conditions and the other under double-blind conditions. In this way the influence of suggestion could have been completely isolated as the independent variable. However, there had been no indication that patients reported symptoms inconsistently. Indeed, we designed the study so that patients were chosen for their consistent selective sensitivity to active injections under unblinded conditions. The physicians had the opportunity to withdraw patients from the study, both after the initial selection and on the day of the testing session. Thus, we must assume that within the range of accuracy of the clinical testing routinely performed in these physicians' offices, the patients were "responders" under unblinded conditions and "nonresponders" under double-blind conditions. We conclude that the technique as practiced works only if practiced unblinded—that is, under the influence of direct or indirect suggestion. This same conclusion can be drawn from a study of symptom-neutralization procedures, in which the rate of symptom relief was independent of the contents of the syringe.[15]

Our study was conducted primarily with provocation doses that were lower than the neutralizing doses. Such "underdoses" were chosen for several reasons. Proponents have asserted that the symptoms provoked by underdoses are stronger, have a more rapid onset, and are somewhat briefer than the symptoms provoked by overdoses. With underdoses, there is less chance of a local skin reaction that would violate the double-blinding. The finding that underdoses provoke symptoms would establish that the dose-symptom curve is not monotonic (that dilutions both greater and less than the neutralizing dose stimulate more intense symptoms than does the neutralizing dose). A dose-symptom curve with a minimal value at the neutralizing dose would justify treatment with the neutralizing dose, since any other dilution would produce more intense symptoms. On the other hand, if underdoses did not provoke symptoms, then there would be no basis for clinically determining the concentration of the neutralizing dose, since underdoses could be used as treatment doses, without concern for the possibility of provoking adverse symptoms. Our results show that underdoses do not provoke symptoms at a rate greater than that for placebo, and that the symptoms do not last significantly longer than those associated with the placebo responses. Thus, in these patients, symptom provocation due to an underdose is not an adequate justification for claiming that treatment with a neutralizing dose is necessary.

It is regrettable that every patient undergoing challenge or provocation testing is not tested in a double-blind fashion, so that the effect of suggestion or anxiety on the end points could be evaluated. If they were so tested, the problems with the validity of the method that we found would have been discovered decades ago. Double-blind testing is easy to incorporate into the routine use of provocation testing or wheal measurements. Indeed, routine practice in standard allergy testing includes the use of diluent tests because sensitivity varies in various parts of the back, and even such standard tests may not be immune to the influence of psychological factors.[18-20] It should be emphasized that double-blind testing is needed not only in clinical medicine but in the physical sciences as well. Langmuir has reviewed several areas in physics in which nonexistent phenomena were the subject of hundreds of papers.[21] These phenomena and provocation testing share the following characteristics: The magnitude of the effect is substantially independent of the intensity of the cause, the effect is close to the limits of detectability, there are claims of great accuracy (or selectivity), and the results are explained by theories that are contrary to common experience.

If the development of the provocation-neutralization technique was determined primarily by placebo responses, then we would expect differences in technique from office to office without a noticeable difference in the outcomes observed by the physicians. This is certainly the case in the current study. Some physicians believed that the best response would be obtained from those who had had little or no treatment, whereas others believed that the patients who had had more treatment were more likely to respond. Similarly, there was disagreement about whether neutralization during the session would affect the subsequent responses in that patient (neutralization after the occurrence of symptoms had no effect on our results). One would have expected some consensus on this issue before our study began if these were not placebo responses, since neutralizing doses are commonly used to relieve acute symptoms, as well as to provide "protection" against subsequent exposure to the substance.

Healing systems without a sound scientific basis flourish in the vacuum created by the inability of modern allopathic medicine to understand or treat many common symptoms. A system of treatment based on the relief of symptoms alone may come to be dominated by placebo reactions. That the field of clinical ecology may have developed disease and treatment concepts based on placebo responses is suggested by the increase in the number of placebo responses that are considered to be symptoms of disease. In 1976, Toogood, quoting Pogge, listed 22 nonspecific symptoms reported in response to the administration of a placebo in 67 clinical studies.[22] Of these 22 symptoms, only 5 were listed as symptoms of food allergy in 1951 by Rinkel and colleagues.[2] Today, 21 of the 22 symptoms commonly seen in response to placebo administration are considered to be indicators of "environmental hypersensitivity," including food sensitivity.

References

1. Lee CH, Williams RI, Binkley EL Jr. Provocative testing and treatment for foods. Arch Otolaryngol 90:87–94, 1969.
2. Rinkel HJ, Lee CH, Brown DW Jr, Willoughby JW, Williams IM. The diagnosis of food allergy. Arch Otolaryngol 79:71–79, 1964.
3. Willoughby IW. Provocative food test technique. Ann Allergy 23:543–554, 1965.
4. Provocative and neutralization testing (subcutaneous). J Allergy Clin Immunol 67:336–337, 1981.
5. Clinical ecology—A critical appraisal. West J Med 144:239–245, 1986.
6. Clinical ecology. J Allergy Clin Immunol 78:269–271, 1986.
7. Crawford LV, Lieberman P, Harfi HA, and others. A double-blind study of subcutaneous food testing sponsored by the Food Committee of the American Academy of Allergy. J Allergy Clin Immunol 57:236, 1976, abstract.
8. Bronsky EA, Burkley DP, Ellis EF. Evaluation of the provocative food skin test technique. J Allergy 47:104, 1971, abstract.
9. Draper WL. Food testing in allergy: Intradermal provocative vs. deliberate feeding. Arch Otolaryngol 95:169–171, 1972.
10. Forman R. A critique of evaluation studies of sublingual and intracutaneous provocative tests for food allergy. Med Hypotheses 7:1019–1027, 1981.
11. King DS. Psychological and behavioral effects of food and chemical exposure in sensitive individuals. Nutr Health 3:137–151, 1984.
12. Fleiss JL. Statistical Methods for Rates and Proportions, Second edition. New York: John Wiley, 1981.
13. Miller JB. Food allergy: Provocative testing and injection therapy. Springfield, Ill.: Charles C Thomas, 1972:7.
14. Hosen H. Clinical Allergy Based on Provocation Testing. Hicksville, N.Y.: Exposition Press, 1978:96.
15. Kailin EW, Collier R. "Relieving" therapy for antigen exposure. JAMA 217:78, 1971.
16. Willoughby JW. Subcutaneous provocative food challenge test. Arch Soc of Clin Ecol 2:102, 1983.
17. Beecher HK. The powerful placebo. JAMA 159:1602–1606, 1955.
18. Black S. Inhibition of immediate-type hypersensitivity response by direct suggestion under hypnosis. BW 1:925–929, 1963.
19. *Idem*. Shift in dose-response curve of Prausnitz-Küstner reaction by direct suggestion under hypnosis. BMJ 1:990–992, 1963.
20. Black S, Humphrey JH, Niven JSF. Inhibition of Mantoux reaction by direct suggestion under hypnosis. BMJ 1:1649–1652, 1963.
21. Langmuir I. Pathological science. Phys Today 42:36–48, 1989.
22. Toogood JH. Perennial rhinitis with negative allergy skin tests. Otorhinolaryngol Dig 38:7, 1976.

Appendix B

Positions of the American Academy of Allergy, Asthma and Immunology

In 1986, the executive committee of the American Academy of Allergy, Asthma and Immunology (then called the American Academy of Allergy and Immunology) issued groundbreaking position statements on clinical ecology, candidiasis hypersensitivity, and the need for proper testing of unproven procedures. The committee members were: John A. Anderson, M.D.; Hyman Chai, M.D.; Henry N. Claman, M.D.; Elliot F. Ellis, M.D.; Jordan N. Fink, M.D.; Allen P. Kaplan, M.D.; Philip L. Lieberman, M.D.; William E. Pierson, M.D.; John E. Salvaggio, M.D.; Albert L. Sheffer, M.D.; and Raymond G. Slavin, M.D. These statements are reproduced from the *Journal of Allergy and Clinical Immunology* 78:269–277, 1986, with permission from Mosby-Year Book, Inc.

CLINICAL ECOLOGY

Background

Clinical ecology is an approach to medicine that ascribes a wide range of symptoms to exposure to numerous common substances in the environment.[1-7] Advocates of this practice describe themselves as "ecologically orientated." Patients are said to be "environmentally ill," or "hypersensitive," or "allergic" to environmental factors such as food, water, chemicals, and pollutants.

It is suggested that this adverse host response and multiple symptomatology develop after prolonged environmental exposure. Once such "sensitivity" has occurred, individuals become sensitive to multiple other environmental exposures (foods, chemicals, etc.). Symptoms exhibited as a result of so-called ecologic disease are multiple. These include behavior disorders, depression, chronic fatigue, arthritis, hypertension, learning disabilities, schizophrenia, gastrointestinal symptoms, respiratory problems, and urinary complaints. There are very few symptoms that have not been considered to be related to such an etiology.

Theron Randolph,[1,3] a founder of the clinical ecology movement, believes that traditional allergy is restricted by definition.[1,5] In his view, each person exists in a dynamic equilibrium with his environment with an adaptation to the environment. When this adaptation becomes deranged, i.e., maladaptation, either acute or chronic illness results. He claims that the primary aim in clinical ecology is the demonstration of etiology, i.e., "the cause-and-effect relationships between given environmental exposures and specifically susceptible persons."

Recently, it has been postulated that these chemical and food sensitivities are related to a malfunction of the immune system that has been termed "immune system dysregulation." This concept has been described as follows:

> Immune system dysregulation can develop over a long period of time and is triggered by a single serious viral infection, major stress, fungi infection, particularly *Candida albicans,* and accumulative exposure to toxic chemicals, even at low levels found in our everyday environment or massive chemical exposure. Immune system dysregulation often remains undiagnosed, however, because many physicians faced with its incredible array of seemingly unrelated symptoms and unfamiliar with the available diagnostic methods, misdiagnose it as stress, psychosomatic disease, or the like. The medications commonly prescribed for these problems may suppress the symptoms to some extent but often further aggravate the problem without dealing with the underlying disease process. When the immune system is malfunctioning, it causes a broad range of symptoms and reaction to a number of harmless or even beneficial substances entering the body. The malfunction commonly originates with the T cells. When the normal complement of T cells are reduced in number or when their ability to function is impaired, they can

no longer adequately control B cell production of antibodies. Without this control, the B cells cannot distinguish harmless dust, pollen, animal dander, or vital and nutritious foods from toxic chemicals or life-threatening bacteria or viruses. The actual healing process from immune system dysregulation is long, slow, and punctuated by exasperating short-term setbacks. These setbacks are part of the healing process and invariably follow a roller coaster pattern. The frequency, duration, and severity of setbacks gradually diminish until symptoms are mild and occur only occasionally.[2]

In establishing a diagnosis for "ecologically related" disease, the testing techniques include serial end point titration and the use of subcutaneous and sublingual provocation and neutralization techniques in addition to RAST and paper radioimmunosorbent tests.[2] Other modalities include fasting, except for water, and introduction of new foods in a cyclic manner. Multiple tests of the immune system are frequently done, including assays of B and T cells, complement, immune complexes, and lymphocyte function.

Treatment usually requires major changes in the home environment and lifestyle. Diets are often highly restricted. Often foods are rotated in a cyclic manner in which a specific food is ingested every three or four days. Processed foods containing coloring or flavoring agents are often eliminated. At times, a total elimination diet, except for special spring waters, is prescribed initially, followed by simple oral challenges with less contaminated organic foods. At times, the patient is hospitalized in a comprehensive environmental control unit in a presumably chemically free environment. Home and working environments are restricted with recommendations for so-called "safe rooms." These are special isolation rooms where the air is filtered and from which all synthetic materials have been removed. Social lives are often markedly restricted, since most environments away from home are "unsafe."

In addition to dietary and environmental restrictions, patients are frequently treated with solutions of "allergens" administered either by injection or sublingually. They are generally low in dosage and follow the provocation and neutralization technique. In addition to the conventional food, pollen, and mold allergens, "immunization" treatment may include chemicals, such as phenol, formaldehyde, histamine, and serotonin.

Critique

The environment is very important in the lives of every human being. Environmental factors, such as chemicals and pollutants, have been demonstrated to influence health. The idea that the environment is responsible for a multitude of human health problems is most appealing. However, to present such ideas as facts, conclusions, or even likely mechanisms without adequate support, is poor medical practice.

The theoretical basis for ecologic illness in the present context has not been established as factual, nor is there satisfactory evidence to support the actual existence of "immune system dysregulation" or maladaptation. There is no clear evidence that many of the symptoms noted above are related to allergy, sensitivity, toxicity, or any other type of reaction from foods, water, chemicals, pollutants, viruses, and bacteria in the context presented. Properly controlled studies defining objective parameters of illness, properly controlled evaluation of the treatment modalities, and appropriate patient assessment have not been done. Anecdotal articles do not constitute sufficient evidence of a cause-and-effect relationship between symptoms and environmental exposure. The major techniques used by the clinical ecologists are controversial and unproven. The American Academy of Allergy and Immunology has previously published position statements concerning subcutaneous and sublingual provocation-neutralization procedures and found them to be unproven.[8] More recent review of new data submitted by a number of clinical ecologists to the Practice Standards Committee of the Academy has not changed that recommendation. There are no adequate studies of the cyclic diets, elimination diets, injection therapy with chemicals, or even the environmentally controlled units to substantiate their use. Many of the patients are reported to have a normal physical examination and normal laboratory tests.

There are no immunologic data to support the dogma of the clinical ecologists. To suggest that these patients lack suppressor T-cell function has not been supported by published data. The suggestion that neutralization therapy can provide rapid relief within minutes or hours cannot be supported by controlled clinical studies or immunologic data.

There does remain the problem of the patient with multiple symptoms who does not clearly fit any disease category and whose illness fails to respond to conventional therapy. These patients are often labeled psychosomatic, a concept that many patients and physicians have trouble accepting and managing. That dilemma may lead the patient to seek out the clinical ecologist. As Brodsky points out:

> This medical subculture (clinical ecology) does not talk about cures; the health-care professionals neither promise nor give hope of eliminating the offending condition, and the patients do not seem to expect it. Like people with diabetes or with long-standing inflammatory bowel disease, they accept the inevitable. In contrast, however, patients seem content with their condition and the reassurance that their symptoms have a physical cause.[9]

Summary

An objective evaluation of the diagnostic and therapeutic principles used to support the concept of clinical ecology indicates that it is an unproven and experimental methodology. It is time-consuming and places severe restrictions on the individual's lifestyle. Individuals who are being treated in this manner should be fully informed of its experimental nature.

Advocates of this dogma should provide adequate clinical and immunologic studies supporting their concepts, which meet the usually accepted standards for scientific investigation.

References

1. Randolph TG. The future of medicine in a monotonous polluted world. Bull Hum Ecol Res Found 1980.
2. Position paper: A new medical specialty designed to identify and treat environmental illness, 1983–1984. Soc Clin Eco.
3. Randolph TG. Graphic representation of clinical ecology. Clin Ecol 2:27, 1983.
4. Randolph TG. Ecologic-orientation in medicine: Comprehensive environmental control in diagnosis and therapy. Ann Allergy 23:7, 1965.
5. Rea WJ, Sell IR, Suits CW, and others. Food and chemical susceptibility after environmental chemical overexposure: Case histories. Ann Allergy 41:101, 1978.
6. Rea WJ. The environmental aspects of ear, nose, and throat disease. Part 1. JCEORL Allergy 41:41, 1979.
7. Mandell M, Conte AA. The role of allergy in arthritis, rheumatism, and polysymptomatic cerebral, visceral, and somatic disorders: A double-blind study. J Intern Acad Prev Med 7, 1982.
8. Reisman RE. American Academy of Allergy. Position statements—controversial techniques. J Allergy Clin Immunol 67:333, 1981.
9. Brodsky CM. "Allergic to everything": A medical subculture. Psychosomatics 24:731, 1983.

CANDIDIASIS HYPERSENSITIVITY SYNDROME

Description

This syndrome has been described and popularized by Truss[1-3] and Crook.[4] The symptoms are described as wide ranging, involving multiple systems, and include fatigue; lethargy; depression; inability to concentrate; hyperactivity; headaches; skin problems, including urticaria; gastrointestinal symptoms such as constipation, abdominal pain, diarrhea, gas and bloating; respiratory tract symptoms; and symptoms involving urinary tract and reproductive organs. Crook[4] recommends to patients:

> Before assuming your symptoms are caused or triggered by the common yeast germ *Candida albicans,* go to your physician for a careful history and physical examination and appropriate laboratory studies or tests. An examination is important because many other disorders can cause similar symptoms. However, if a careful checkup doesn't reveal the cause for your symptoms and your medical history [as described in this book] is "typical," it's possible or even probable that your health problems are yeast connected [page 11].

He further notes that tests do not help much because:

> *Candida* germs live in every person's body—especially on the mucous membranes. Accordingly, vaginal and other smears and cultures for *Candida* don't help. Therefore the diagnosis is suspected from the patient's history and confirmed by his response to treatment[4] [pages 27, 28].

The alleged basis for the syndrome is described by Crook as follows:

> Antibiotics, especially broad spectrum antibiotics, kill "friendly germs" while they're killing enemies. And when friendly germs are knocked out, yeast germs *(Candida albicans)* multiply. Diets rich in carbohydrates and yeasts, birth control pills, cortisone, and other drugs also stimulate yeast growth. Large numbers of yeasts weaken your immune system. Your immune system is also affected adversely by nutritional deficiencies, sugar consumption, and by exposure to environmental molds and chemicals (such as formaldehyde, petrochemicals, perfume, and tobacco). When your immune system is compromised and your resistance is lessened, you may feel bad "all over" and develop

respiratory, digestive, and other symptoms. And you're apt to develop adverse reactions to additional foods, inhalants, and chemicals. As a part of these reactions, mucous membranes throughout your body swell, and you develop infections caused by bacteria and viruses that a strong immune system would ordinarily conquer. When you develop an infection, you're apt to be given "broad spectrum" antibiotics. Such antibiotics, while at times essential, promote the growth of *Candida albicans* which depress your immune system. And your health problems continue until the vicious cycle is interrupted by a comprehensive treatment program designed to decrease the growth of *Candida albicans* and increase your resistance[4] [pages 15, 16].

The recommended program for the candidiasis hypersensitivity syndrome includes:

1. Continuing observation in order that concomitant diseases can be detected, accurately diagnosed, and specifically treated.
2. Exercise program.
3. Mental health program.
4. Avoidance of chemical pollutants.
5. Use of antioxidants.
6. Use of special laboratory tests:
   a. Ratio of helper cells to suppressor cells.
   b. Blood vitamin studies.
   c. Mineral studies in hair, blood, and urine.
   d. Amino acid studies in urine.
   e. Essential fatty acid profile.
7. Special dietary program:
   a. Diet nutritionally adequate with fresh foods from a variety of sources.
   b. Diversified diet.
   c. Avoidance of all refined carbohydrates, including sugar, corn syrup, dextrose, and fructose.
   d. Avoid refined, processed, and fabricated foods.
   e. Avoid fruits and milk initially. Later, try to rotate fruits back into the diet if they are tolerated.
   f. Avoid all yeast and mold-containing foods initially. Ultimately, some of these may prove to be tolerated, since a yeast-containing food does not make *Candida albicans* organisms grow.
   g. Eat sugar-free yogurt.

    h. Take nutritional supplements, including vitamins, minerals, and essential fatty acids.
8. Use of antifungal agents:
    a. Nystatin.
    b. Clotrimazole.
    c. Ketoconazole (Nizoral).
    d. Amphotericin B.
    These agents may be used orally or topically in the vagina for months.
9. Use of allergenic extracts of *Candida albicans* for
    a. immunotherapy and/or
    b. provocation/neutralization.

Dr. Crook emphasizes two points about his program for candidiasis hypersensitivity syndrome that are of great importance:

a. The disorder is very common and has multiple manifestations. Any physician who reads his book will recognize that patients with the complaints described are very common indeed.

b. The disorder can be diagnosed only by favorable response to his treatment program administered over a sufficient period of time. He emphasizes that treatment requires time, patience, persistence, and careful management of the multiple factors contributing to the illness.

Critique

The Practice Standards Committee finds multiple problems with the candidiasis hypersensitivity syndrome.

1. The concept is speculative and unproven.
    a. The basic elements of the syndrome would apply to almost all sick patients at some time. The complaints are essentially universal; the broad treatment program (see Description of Syndrome, particularly elements 1, 2, 3, and 7a) would produce remission in most illnesses regardless of cause.
    b. There is no published proof that *Candida albicans* is responsible for the syndrome.
    c. There is no published proof that treatment of *Candida albicans* infection with specific antifungal agents (see Description 8) benefits the syndrome.

d. There is no proof that immunotherapy or provocation and/or neutralization with *Candida albicans* allergenic extracts (see Description 9) benefit the syndrome.

e. There is no proof that the recommended special studies (see Description 6) are effective diagnostic tests for the purposes for which they are used.

2. Elements of the proposed treatment program are potentially dangerous.

a. Resistant species of *Candida albicans* and of other pathogenic fungi may be produced by long-term oral use of the major antifungal agents (see Description 8).

b. Untoward effects from oral use of antifungal agents (see Description 8) are rare, but some inevitably will occur.

Recommendations

On the basis of the evidence so far reviewed and until appropriate published evidence to the contrary is brought to its attention, the Practice Standards Committee recommends that the concept of the candidiasis hypersensitivity syndrome (see Description of Syndrome) is unproven. The diagnosis, the special laboratory tests (see Description of Syndrome 6), and the special aspects of treatment (see Description of Syndrome 8 and 9) should be considered experimental and reserved for use with informed consent in appropriate controlled trials that have been approved for scientific merit and safety by competent institutional review boards.

References

1. Truss CO. Tissue injury induced by *Candida albicans:* Mental and neurologic manifestations. J Orthomolecular Psychiatry 7:17, 1978.
2. Truss CO. Restoration of immunologic competence to *Candida albicans.* J Orthomolecular Psychiatry 9:287, 1980.
3. Truss CO. The role of *Candida albicans* in human illness. J Orthomolecular Psychiatry 10:228, 1981.
4. Crook WG. The Yeast Connection: A Medical Breakthrough, 2nd ed. Jackson, Tenn.: Professional Books, 1984.

UNPROVEN PROCEDURES FOR DIAGNOSIS AND TREAT-MENT OF ALLERGIC AND IMMUNOLOGIC DISEASES

Definition of an Unproven Procedure

An unproven procedure for the diagnosis and treatment of allergic and immunologic diseases is defined as any specific procedure for these purposes that has not been proven effective by proper trial.

Recommended Policy for Processing an Unproven Procedure

All newly proposed procedures are unproven when they are first introduced. The future of the field of allergy and immunology and of the patient with allergic and immunologic diseases will be strongly influenced by the care with which these unproven procedures are developed and tested by those who initiate and sponsor them. The unproven procedure should be subjected to a fair trial to determine whether or not it is effective, the circumstances under which it is effective, and its relative merit with reference to other effective procedures for the same purpose. During the trial period, the procedure should be considered experimental and reserved for use with informed consent in appropriate controlled trials that have been approved for safety and scientific merit by competent institutional review boards. The procedure should not be accepted for general use until proof of effectiveness has been established and published in reputable "refereed" medical journals. Procedures that have not been proven effective may continue to be used on an experimental basis as described above or discarded but should not be sanctioned for routine use. Unless a physician is concerned with the trial, a physician or a medical facility should have no obligation to use the procedure or to transmit knowledge of it.

An unproven procedure can be proven effective, since it is possible to prove a positive point. However, under most circumstances, it is not possible to prove that a procedure is ineffective, because one cannot prove a negative point. Therefore, the biomedical community should require proof of effectiveness of a procedure before the procedure is accepted for routine use but should not demand proof of ineffectiveness before discarding the unproven procedure.

The responsibility for testing the unproven procedure should rest with the proponent of the procedure, since the proponent understands and favors the procedure and can make sure that the trial is a proper one. The responsibility for reviewing the plans for and the results of the trial should reside with at least four groups of peers: (1) physicians who work with and know the proponent, (2) the institutional review board that reviews the trial protocol for safety and scientific merit, (3) the editorial board and critics selected by the editorial board of the journal that considers for publication the manuscript that represents the recorded results of the trial, and (4) appointed practice standards committees of allergy specialty societies such as the Practice Standards Committee of the American Academy of Allergy and Immunology. Each of these four groups of peers should on request by the proponent or other interested party provide a written critique of the recorded proposals for and accomplishments of the trial. Institutional review boards should have primary responsibility for proposals, editorial boards for unpublished reports of accomplishments, and practice standard committees for published reports of accomplishments.

Necessity for Proper Trials

There is considerable evidence that indicates that neither patient nor physician can distinguish between an effective and an ineffective procedure without performing a proper trial. For example, before controlled trials, for at least 40 years, low-dose immunotherapy with ragweed pollen extract was considered to be effective treatment for ragweed hay fever. In recent years, a number of controlled trials have indicated that low-dose immunotherapy was no more effective than placebos,[2-5] whereas immunotherapy with large doses of ragweed extract was effective,[3,5,6-11] was specific for ragweed hay fever,[3,9] and induced immunologic changes not induced by low-dose immunotherapy or placebo that included an increase in protective IgG antibody to ragweed,[3,5,11-15] an initial increase in specific IgE antibody,[3,5,11-14] a diminution of the expected seasonal rise in IgE antibody to ragweed,[3,5,10-14] and an ultimate decrease in ragweed IgE toward pretreatment levels.[3,12,14] Nevertheless, many patients who received low-dose immunotherapy or placebos were of the opinion that they had received an effective treatment.[4,5,11]

Before controlled trials, for more than 10 years, whole body extract of various Hymenoptera insects such as honeybees, yellow jackets, hornets, and wasps were used to diagnose and treat anaphylactic reaction to their stings. Both patients and physicians were of the opinion that these extracts were effective for both diagnosis and therapy.[16] In recent years, a series of controlled trials comparing the effects of Hymenoptera venoms, Hymenoptera whole body extracts, and placebos have demonstrated that immunotherapy with whole body extracts was no more effective than placebos, whereas venoms were clearly effective.[16] Furthermore, the controlled trials demonstrated that skin tests with Hymenoptera venoms were effective for distinguishing patients with a history of anaphylactic reactions to Hymenoptera stings from nonallergic patients, whereas skin tests with Hymenoptera whole body extracts were not effective for this purpose.[16]

Proper Trials

A proper trial of an unproven procedure for diagnosis and therapy of allergic and immunologic diseases must deal effectively with problems that derive from the fact that the manifestations of these diseases in different patients run various courses that depend on a number of extrinsic factors that include allergens, emotional tension, irritants, infection, and/or intrinsic factors such as the severity of the patient's sensitivity to allergens. The design of the trial should permit the investigator to separate the effects of the procedure being tested from the effects of other factors. The hypothesis to be tested should be stated clearly and related precisely to previously established fact and to its scientific basis. Reagents and procedures should be described and used in such a way that they could be used in similar manner by subsequent investigators. They should not be used in the trial until they are developed to a point where they elicit consistent results under standard circumstances. The trial should concern a homogeneous group of patients whose characteristics are well described in order that similar patients could be found by a subsequent investigator. These patients should have the abnormality under study but otherwise be essentially well. Such patients may not be found easily in the practices or allergy clinics of the investigators, and recruitment by advertisement in the media may be necessary. These patients should be stratified with reference to risk factors that might modify response, such as sensitivity to allergen. Then, by random selection, they should be divided into groups of equal size in such a fashion that patients in each study group have comparable characteristics and risk factors. By random selection, study groups should be assigned to test and control procedures. Results of the procedure should be evaluated as objectively as possible and expressed in quantifiable terms. If evaluation depends on a patient's or physician's judgment, the trial should be conducted "double-blind" in order that neither patient nor evaluating physicians know which patient received a specific test or control procedure. Appropriate statistical methods for evaluating the results of the study should be selected at the time of design of the study.

It is evident that before controlled trials were done, worthless procedures for diagnosis and therapy of allergic and immunologic diseases have been accepted as effective by both patient and physician. Therefore, proper trials are necessary, and an unproven procedure should be considered to be experimental and likely to be ineffective until proven to be effective.

Recommendations

The science of allergy and immunology has advanced to the point where effective procedures for diagnosis and treatment of allergic and immunologic diseases can be proven to be effective. Currently available procedures of proven effectiveness are sufficiently satisfactory for diagnosis and treatment of allergic and immunologic diseases so that procedures of unproven effectiveness should not be used in routine fashion but rather should be considered experimental and reserved for use with informed consent in controlled trials that have been approved for safety and scientific merit by competent and institutional review boards.

References

1. Lowell FC. Some untested diagnostic and therapeutic procedures in clinical allergy. J Allergy Clin Immunol 56:168, 1975.
2. Hirsch SR. Kalbfleisch JH, Golbert TM, and others. Rinkel injection therapy: A multicenter controlled study. J Allergy Clin Immunol 68:133, 1981.
3. Norman PS. Immunotherapy. Prog Allergy 32:318, 1982.

4. Van Metre TE, Adkinson NF, Lichtenstein LM, Mardiney MR, Norman PS, Rosenberg GL, Sobotka AK, Valentine MD. A controlled study of the effectiveness of the Rinkel method of immunotherapy for ragweed pollen hay fever. J Allergy Clin Immunol 65:288, 1980.

5. Van Metre TE, Adkinson NF, Amodio FJ, Lichtenstein LM, Mardiney MR, Norman PS, Rosenberg GL, Sobotka AK, Valentine MD. A comparative study of the effectiveness of the Rinkel method and of the current standard method of immunotherapy for ragweed pollen hay fever. J Allergy Clin Immunol 66:500, 1980.

6. Franklin W, Lowell FC. Comparison of two dosages of ragweed extract in the treatment of pollenosis. JAMA 201:915, 1967.

7. Hirsch SR, Kalbfleisch JH, Cohen SH. Comparison of Rinkel injection therapy with standard immunotherapy. J Allergy Clin Immunol 70:183, 1982.

8. Lowell FC, Franklin W. A "double-blind" study of treatment with aqueous allergenic extracts in cases of allergic rhinitis. J Allergy Clin Immunol 34:165, 1963.

9. Lowell FC, Franklin W. A double-blind study of the effectiveness and specificity of injection therapy in ragweed hay fever. N Engl J Med 273:675, 1965.

10. Norman PS, Lichtenstein LM, Ishizaka K. Diagnostic tests in ragweed hay fever: A comparison of direct skin tests, IgE antibody measurements, and basophil histamine release. J Allergy Clin Immunol 52:210, 1973.

11. Van Metre TE, Adkinson NF, Amodio FJ, Lichtenstein LM, Mardiney MR, Norman PS, Rosenberg GL, Sobotka AK, Valentine MD. A comparison of immunotherapy schedules for injection treatment of ragweed pollen hay fever. J Allergy Clin Immunol 69:181, 1982.

12. Creticos PS, Van Metre TE, Mardiney MR, Rosenberg GL, Norman PS, Adkinson NF. Dose response of IgE and IgG antibodies during ragweed immunotherapy. J Allergy Clin Immunol 73:94, 1984.

13. Gleich GJ, Jacob GL, Yunginger JW, Henderson LL. Measurement of the absolute levels of IgE antibodies in patients with ragweed hay fever: Effect of immunotherapy on seasonal changes and relationship to IgG antibodies. J Allergy Clin Immunol 60:188, 1977.

14. Gleich GJ, Zimmerman EM, Henderson LL, Yunginger JW. Effect of immunotherapy on immunoglobulin E and immunoglobulin G antibodies to ragweed antigens: A six-year prospective study. J Allergy Clin Immunol 70:261, 1982.

15. Irons JS, Pruzansky JJ, Patterson R, Zeiss CR. Studies of perennial ragweed immunotherapy, associated changes in cellular responsiveness, total serum antigen-binding capacity, and specific IgE antibody concentrations. J Allergy Clin Immunol 59:190, 1977.

16. Lichtenstein LM, Valentine MD, Sobotka AK. Insect allergy: The state of the art. J Allergy Clin Immunol 64:5, 1979.

Appendix C

Clinical Ecology: Position Statement of the American Medical Association

Physicians who practice clinical ecology believe that exposure to low levels of environmental substances present in the air or ingested from food and liquids causes in susceptible individuals a variety of ill-defined symptoms affecting nearly every organ system.

Multiple Chemical Sensitivity Syndrome

Most physicians who practice clinical ecology (clinical ecologists) maintain that a number of patients have the multiple chemical sensitivity syndrome (MCSS) (also called clinical ecological illness, environmental illness, chemical AIDS [acquired immunodeficiency syndrome], 20th-Century disease, environmental hypersensitivity disease, total allergy syndrome, and cerebral allergy).[1-10] Clinical ecology has been defined as the orientation in medicine in which physicians primarily work with patients to uncover the cause-and-effect relationship between their ill health and food or low-level chemical exposure.[9] Other definitions have been offered and no general agreement exists that clinical ecology and MCSS are synonymous.[8-10] The lack of a clear definition or diagnostic test for MCSS has made it difficult to estimate its prevalence in the United States.

From the AMA Council on Scientific Affairs. Reprinted with permission from JAMA 268:3465–3467, 1992. Copyright 1992, American Medical Association.

Clinical ecologists report that significant numbers of people have immune system derangements that increase their sensitivity to low levels of substances in the environment that are innocuous to normal people and are either inhaled (e.g., the outside air, the workplace, or home) or ingested as liquids, foods, or drugs.[4-6] Exposure to such substances in susceptible individuals is alleged to produce a polysymptomatic disorder that may involve any organ or many organ systems. Predisposing risk factors are said to include infection due to *Candida albicans,* a deficient or inadequate diet, and/or food intolerance. The primary complaints of such patients include allergy-like symptoms, food and chemical intolerance, rhinitis, difficulty in breathing, depression, headache, fatigue, irritability, insomnia, palpitations, and other cardiovascular symptoms.

A subset of MCSS is the *Candida* hypersensitivity syndrome.[7] Some patients fit the criteria for chronic fatigue syndrome (CFS).[11] Multiple chemical sensitivity is also claimed to be a cause or a contributing factor in the development of a number of recognized diseases and disorders (e.g., migraine, various psychiatric illnesses, urticaria, anaphylaxis, atopic dermatitis, allergic rhinitis, asthma, learning disabilities, arthritis, and susceptibility to cancer).

Clinical ecologists propose a series of events to explain the development of MCSS. Low concentrations of a number of different chemicals over time are purported to damage the immune system and produce symptoms and sensitivity to other substances. The total load (body burden) of environmental insult is considered critical for the induction of illness. The concept of total load was introduced to explain inconsistent development of symptoms and variable dose-response findings after experimental exposure to chemicals and food.[3,12,13] Changes in the frequency of exposure and intervals between exposures to a specific antigen may delay the onset of symptoms and alter the sensitivity of a patient to the offending substance.[12] Clinical ecologists report that unrecognized immune system dysregulation develops over a long period after cumulative exposure to certain chemicals. Further, overt manifestations are purported to be triggered by a single serious viral infection, major stress, or fungal infection (particularly *C albicans*). One currently popular hypothesis suggests that damage to T cells by chemicals or other agents causes inversion of the normal helper/suppressor T-cell ratio, and as a result alters antibody production by B cells.[10] To assess immune dysfunction, some investigators have reported that analysis of

T- and B-cell surface markers and assay of a variety of specific antibodies (e.g., formaldehyde and isocyanates) could be useful in diagnostic testing.[10]

Therapeutic Approaches

Avoidance is a major aspect of therapy; patients are often told to ingest a defined or restricted diet or use a rotation diet, to move to another location, to create an environmentally "safe" room in their home, or in severe cases to be placed temporarily in special environmental isolation units (such units are used primarily for investigational purposes and are rarely used for treatment).

A major technique used by many practitioners of clinical ecology is sublingual or intradermal provocation-neutralization. It is used for diagnostic purposes (provocation) or for therapy to relieve symptoms (neutralization). With this procedure, a diluted extract of the suspected antigen is administered sublingually or intradermally. The prompt development of symptoms confirms the substance as causative. Once the dose that elicits symptoms has been determined, decreasing doses of the antigen are administered until symptoms disappear; this is the neutralization dose.[14-20] The mechanisms for these effects are unknown. Although a large number of uncontrolled studies have been conducted and a large body of anecdotal evidence is available, no well-controlled studies have demonstrated either diagnostic or therapeutic value for provocation-neutralization.[1-3,6] In one recent double-blind trial of provocation-neutralization, a placebo was as effective as injection of food extracts to induce either symptoms or neutralization.[21] In contrast, two other studies supported the value of these techniques for diagnosis and treatment.[22,23] These three studies and other reports[14-20] have been criticized for design and methodologic flaws.

Two models have been reported that might permit controlled studies of provocation-neutralization.[24-28]

Candida Hypersensitivity Syndrome

Many clinical ecologists believe that the fungus *Candida albicans is* a major cause of symptoms associated with MCSS.[7,29] It is claimed that repeated use of antibiotics, birth control pills, corticosteroids, and/or an improper or defective diet can lead to overgrowth and a systemic infection by this organism. Clinical ecologists also claim that *C albicans* produces a toxin or other substances that disrupt bowel chemistry and immune function in susceptible patients. However, *Candida is* a constituent of the normal gastrointestinal tract in many healthy individuals. Because reliable tests to detect *Candida* or its putative toxin systemically in levels postulated to exist by clinical ecologists are unavailable, diagnosis is by exclusion and the only proof of *Candida*-related disease is response to therapy. Although considerable anecdotal evidence supports the existence of *Candida* hypersensitivity syndrome through its response to therapy with antifungal agents, nutritional supplements, and dietary manipulation, scientific proof from well-controlled studies has not been provided.[30-34]

Chronic Fatigue Syndrome

Considerable controversy exists over whether this alleged syndrome is a specific disease entity. Patients diagnosed as having CFS suffer from a disabling weakness and exhaustion that may continue for months or even years. Some patients lose the ability to think clearly, to concentrate, and to retain memory; confusion, depression, insomnia, and/or hypersomnia often are present. Flu-like symptoms also may be present and include sore throat, headache, fever, and muscle/joint pain. Diagnostic criteria for this syndrome have been proposed.[35] However, no definitive laboratory tests exist. No single cause for this syndrome appears likely.[8,11,36-38]

An infectious or immunological mechanism has been investigated with few tangible results. In particular, suggestions have been made that infection (e.g., Epstein-Barr virus, human herpesvirus 6, human T-cell leukemia virus II [HTLV-II], or other environmental insults [e.g., chemicals]) may stimulate cells involved in the immune response and trigger cytokines such as interferon or interleukin 2 as well as other endogenous inflammatory mediators. In a well-controlled study, evidence was presented for the presence of serum antibodies to HTLV-II, a retrovirus, by Western blot in patients with CFS.[39] This finding awaits confirmation by other laboratories. Another well-controlled study demonstrates activation of cytotoxic CDS cells in up to 50% of patients with CFS.[40]

More than two-thirds of patients with CFS appear to have an associated psychiatric disorder.[11,38] Management is difficult although depression and other psychiatric disorders may be treated with drugs and/or psychotherapy. Other treatment is symptomatic and generally not helpful.[11,38]

Sick Building Syndrome

Air quality is poor in many newly constructed buildings, and low levels of toxic agents, allergens, chemicals, or contamination with microorganisms circulating in a closed environment can produce a building-related illness for which a causative agent can be identified (e.g., Legionnaires' disease, humidifier fever, hypersensitivity pneumonia, and building-related asthma). In contrast to building-related illness, no specific causative agent has been identified for the symptoms occurring in patients with the sick building syndrome.[41,42] Symptoms reported in patients with the sick building syndrome include chest tightness, fatigue, headache, malaise, and cough, as well as eye and mucous membrane irritation. The MCSS should not be confused with the sick building syndrome.

The lack of agreement by workers in this field over the definition of the sick building syndrome and inclusion and exclusion criteria for patients suspected of having this syndrome has hampered efforts to design well-controlled studies. Evidence that this syndrome exists as a separate disease entity is weak. Some have claimed that mass hysteria and other psychosocial factors are responsible for symptoms. A few reports discuss building-related illness and the sick building syndrome and provide a basis for studying the latter.[42,43]

Assessment of Clinical Ecology

Validation of MCSS is complicated by the number and variety of symptoms and the lack of objective signs, and by the overlapping of symptoms in a number of alleged clinical ecological illnesses (e.g.,

Candida hypersensitivity and CFS) with those of recognized orders (e.g., depression and polymyalgia rheumatica). The proposed immune imbalance associated with MCSS has not been identified. No evidence based on well-controlled clinical trials is available that supports a cause-and-effect relationship between exposure to very low levels of substances and the myriad symptoms purported by clinical ecologists to result from such exposure. Several articles and books are available that seek to provide a scientific basis for such an association.[7,10,44] Such publications, while thought-provoking and interesting, fail to provide proof based on well-controlled clinical studies.

The view that some patients are allergic to or intolerant of environmental substances is not in itself controversial. Rarely, some individuals are known to be hypersensitive to minute concentrations of a food, drug, or inhalant allergen causing objective illness; on the other hand, clinical ecologists claim that such occurrences are common and not rare and that manifestations are subjective only. Controversy revolves around the minimum concentration of the offending substance that causes adverse reactions, the nature of such adverse effects, and the mechanisms involved.

Although malingering or hypochondriasis may be responsible for symptoms, such a cause appears unlikely in most patients. A number of clinicians have reported that the majority of patients have a definite psychosomatic disorder that could be responsible for symptoms.[32,45-49]

The fact that the diagnostic tests and therapy recommended by clinical ecologists are largely unproven by controlled clinical studies does not necessarily establish the lack of scientific validity. Well-controlled studies could validate and provide a scientific basis for many of the tests and therapies associated with multiple chemical sensitivity. Attempts to design and carry out such controlled studies have been discussed at a recent two-day National Academy of Sciences workshop, a Canadian environmental workshop, in a recent book, and in review articles.[9,10,50,51]

Conclusions

Some patients present to physicians with symptoms that cannot be attributed to any known condition, disorder, or disease. Further, they may have no physical findings or laboratory abnormalities to support a standard diagnosis. The constellation of symptoms presented (e.g., depression, fatigue, irritability, difficulty in breathing, headache, gastrointestinal distress, and food intolerance) resemble those seen in many illnesses. Physicians who practice clinical ecology associate these symptoms with repeated exposure of susceptible individuals to very low levels of substances that exist in the environment or are ingested as food or liquids. After these substances have accumulated to a threshold concentration in the body, they are purported to produce immune dysfunction and result in a generalized clinical disorder—MCSS. Subsets of this syndrome include *Candida* hypersensitivity syndrome and CFS. Some patients diagnosed as having MCSS have an associated psychiatric disorder that could be responsible for many of the symptoms. Other patients are presumed to have a physical basis for symptoms that result from an unrecognized or undefined organic disorder.

Two medical societies have issued position papers and one has issued an informational report on clinical ecology.[1-3] The position papers reported that no scientific evidence supports the contention that MCSS is a significant cause of disease or that the diagnostic tests and the treatments used have any therapeutic value.[1,3] Until such accurate, reproducible, and well-controlled studies are available, the American Medical Association Council on Scientific Affairs believes that multiple chemical sensitivity should not be considered a recognized clinical syndrome.

Based on the reports in the peer-reviewed scientific literature, the Council on Scientific Affairs finds that at this time (1) there are no well-controlled studies establishing a clear mechanism or cause for MCSS; and (2) there are no well-controlled studies providing confirmation of the efficacy of the diagnostic and therapeutic modalities relied on by those who practice clinical ecology.

Recommendations

The Council on Scientific Affairs recognizes that the above findings are those existing at one point in time, and welcomes the opportunity to review well-controlled studies as they become available. It recommends the following:

1. That the American Medical Association continue to monitor the published literature on clinical ecology and report on it as appropriate.

2. That those who support a new test, procedure, or treatment must prove by appropriately controlled peer-reviewed trials that it is effective for the purposes for which it is used and that the burden should not be shifted to opponents to prove that a new test or therapy is invalid.

Background History of Report

This report was presented to the House of Delegates as Report K of the Council on Scientific Affairs at the American Medical Association's interim meeting in December 1991. The recommendation was adopted as amended in lieu of Substitute Resolution 6 (I-90) and the remainder of the report was filed.

This report was not intended to be construed or to serve as a standard of medical care. Standards of medical care are determined on the basis of all the facts and circumstances involved in an individual case and are subject to change as scientific knowledge and technology advance and patterns of practice evolve. This report reflects the views of scientific literature as of December 1991.

The members of the AMA Council on Scientific Affairs were: Yank D. Coble, Jr., M.D., Jacksonville, Fla., Vice-Chairman; E. Harvey Estes, Jr., M.D., Durham, N.C., Chairman; C. Alvin Head, M.D., Tucker, Ga., Resident Representative; Mitchell S. Karlan, M.D., Beverly Hills, Calif.; William R. Kennedy, M.D., Minneapolis, Minn.; Patricia Joy Numann, M.D., Syracuse, N.Y.; William C. Scott, M.D., Tucson, Ariz.; W. Douglas Skelton, M.D., Macon, Ga.; Richard M. Steinhilber, M.D., Cleveland, Ohio; Jack P. Strong, M.D., New Orleans, La.; Christine C. Toevs, Greenville, N.C., Medical Student Representative; Henry N. Wagner, Jr., M.D., Baltimore, Md.; Jerod M. Loeb, Ph.D., Chicago, Ill., Secretary; Robert C. Rinaldi, Ph.D., Chicago, Ill., Assistant Secretary; Steven J. Smith, Ph.D., Chicago, Ill., staff author.

References

1. American Academy of Allergy and Immunology. American Academy of Allergy and Immunology position statement: Clinical ecology. J Allergy Clin Immunol 78:269–271, 1986.
2. Task Force on Clinical Ecology, California Medical Association Scientific Board. Clinical ecology: A critical appraisal. West J Med 144:239–245, 1986.
3. American College of Physicians. American College of Physicians position statement: Clinical ecology. Ann Intern Med 111:168–178, 1989.
4. Randolph TG, Moss RW. An Alternative Approach to Allergies: The New Field of Clinical Ecology Unravels the Environmental Causes of Mental and Physical Ills. New York: Lippincott and Cromwell, 1980.
5. Levin AS, Byers VS. Environmental illness: A disorder of immune regulation. Occup Med 2:669–681, 1987.
6. Black DW, Rathe A. Total environmental allergy: 20th century disease or deception? Resident Staff Physician 36:47–54, 1990.
7. Crook WG. The Yeast Connection, Third edition. Jackson, Tenn.: Professional Books, 1989.
8. Salvaggio JE. Clinical and immunologic approach to patients with alleged environmental injury. Ann Allergy 66:493–503, 1991.
9. Hileman B. Multiple chemical sensitivity. Chem Eng News 69:26–42, July 1991.
10. Ashford NA, Miller CS. Chemical Exposures: Low Levels and High Stakes. New York: Van Nostrand Reinhold Co., 1991.
11. Kroenke K. Chronic fatigue syndrome: Is it real? Postgrad Med 89:44–55, 1991.
12. Bell IR. Clinical ecology. In A New Medical Approach to Environmental Illness. Bolinas, Calif.: Common Knowledge Press, 1982.
13. Rea NJ, Bell JR, Suits CW, Smiley RE. Food and chemical susceptibility after environmental chemical overexposure: Case histories. Ann Allergy 41:101–109, 1978.
14. Council on Scientific Affairs, American Medical Association. In vivo diagnostic testing and immunotherapy for allergy: Report I, part II, of the allergy panel. JAMA 258:1505–1508, 1987.
15. Lee CH. A new test for diagnosis and treatment of food allergies. Med Bull 25:9–12, 1961.
16. Lee CH, Williams RI, Binkley EL. Provocative inhalant testing and treatment. Arch Otolaryngol Head Neck Surg 90:173–177, 1969.
17. Rinkel HJ, Lee CH, Brown DW, Willoughby JW, Williams JM. The diagnosis of food allergy. Arch Otolaryngol Head Neck Surg 79:71–80, 1964.
18. Willoughby JW. Provocative food test technique. Ann Allergy 23:543–554, 1965.

19. Missal SC. Food allergy in eye, ear, nose and throat disease. Otolaryngol Clin North Am 4:479–490, 1971.

20. Miller JB. Food Allergy: Provocative Testing and Injection Therapy. Springfield, Ill.: Charles C Thomas Publishers, 1982.

21. Jewett DL, Fein G, Greenberg MH. A double-blind study of symptom provocation to determine food sensitivity. N Engl J Med 323:429–433, 1989.

22. King WP, Rubin WA, Fadal RG, and others. Provocation-neutralization: A two-part study, part I: The intracutaneous provocative food test: A multicenter comparison study. Otolaryngol Head Neck Surg 99:263–269, 1988.

23. King WP, Fadal RG, Ward WA, and others. Provocation-neutralization: A two-part study, part II: Subcutaneous neutralization therapy: A multicenter study. Otolaryngol Head Neck Surg 99:272–277, 1988.

24. Boris M, Schiff M, Weindorf S, and others. Bronchoprovocation blocked by neutralization therapy. J Allergy Clin Immunol 71:92, 1983. Abstract.

25. Boris M, Weindorf S, Corriel RN, Inselman LS, Schiff M. Antigen induced asthma attenuated by neutralization therapy. Clin Ecology 3:59–62, 1985.

26. Schiff M, Boris M, Weindorf S. Injection of low dose antigen attenuates the response to subsequent bronchoprovocative challenge with the same antigen. Am Rev Respir Dis 131(suppl, pt 2):A38, 1985. Abstract.

27. Boris M, Schiff M, Weindorf S. Injection of low dose antigen attenuates the response to subsequent bronchoprovocative challenge. Otolaryngol Head Neck Surg 98:539–545, 1988.

28. Seadding GK, Brostoff J. Low dose sublingual therapy in patients with allergic rhinitis due to house dust mite. Clin Allergy 16:483–491, 1986.

29. Truss CO. The Missing Diagnosis. Second edition. Birmingham, Ala.: CO Truss, 1986.

30. Renfro L, Feder HM Jr, Lane TJ, Manu P, Matthews DA. Yeast connection among 100 patients with chronic fatigue. Am J Med 86:165–168, 1989.

31. Dismukes WE, Wade JS, Lee JY, Doekery BK, Hain JD. A randomized, double-blind trial of nystatin therapy for the candidiasis hypersensitivity syndrome. N Engl J Med 323:1717–1723, 1990.

32. Black DW, Rathe A, Goldstein RB. Environmental illness: a controlled study of 26 subjects with '20th century disease.' JAMA 264:3166–3170, 1990.

33. Bennett JE. Searching for the yeast connection. N Engl J Med 323:1766–1767, 1990.

34. American Academy of Allergy and Immunology. American Academy of Allergy and Immunology position statement: Candidiasis hypersensitivity syndrome. J Allergy Clin Immunol 78:271–273, 1986.

35. Holmes GP, Kaplan JE, Gantz NM, and others. Chronic fatigue syndrome: A working case definition. Ann Intern Med 108:387–389, 1988.

36. Swartz MN. The chronic fatigue syndrome: One entity or many? N Engl J Med 319:1726–1728, 1988.

37. Gold D, Bowden R, Sixbey J, and others. Chronic fatigue: A prospective clinical and virologic study. JAMA 264:48–53, 1990.

38. Shafran SD. The chronic fatigue syndrome. Am J Med 90:730–739, 1991.

39. DeFreitas E, Hilliard B, Cheney PR, and others. Retroviral sequences related to human T-lymphotrophic virus type II in patients with chronic fatigue immune dysfunction syndrome. Proc Natl Acad Sci USA 88:2922–2926, 1991.

40. Landay AL, Jessop C, Lennette ET, Levy JA. Chronic fatigue syndrome: Clinical condition associated with immune activation. Lancet 338:707–712, 1991.

41. Bardana EJ Jr, Montanaro A, O'Hollaren MT. Building-related illness. Clin Rev Allergy. 6:61–89, 1988.

42. Bardana EJ Jr. Building-related illness. In Bardana EJ Jr., Montanaro A, O'Hollaren HT, editors. Occupational Asthma. Philadelphia, Pa.: Hanley and Belfus, 1991:1–18.

43. Hodgson MJ, Frohliger J, Permar E, and others. Symptoms and microenvironmental measures in nonproblem buildings. J Occup Med 33:527–533, 1991.

44. Cullen MR. The worker with multiple chemical sensitivities: An overview. Occup Med 2:655–661, 1989.

45. Stewart DE, Raskin J. Psychiatric assessment of patients with '20th century disease' ('total allergy syndrome'). Can Med Assoc J 133:1001–1006, 1985.

46. Terr AI. Environmental illness: A clinical review of 50 Cases. Arch Intern Med 146:145–149, 1986.

47. Terr AI. Multiple chemical sensitivities immunologic critique: Clinical ecology theories and practice. Occup Med 2:683–694, 1987.

48. Brodsky CM. Allergic to everything: A medical subculture. Psychosomatics 24:731–742, 1983.

49. Pearson DJ, Rix KJB, Bentley SJ. Food allergy: How much in the mind? A clinical and psychiatric study of suspected food hypersensitivity. Lancet 1:1259–1261, 1983.

50. Hileman B. Chemical sensitivity: Experts agree on research protocol. Chem Eng News 69:4–5, April 1991.

51. Davies JW, Wilkins K, editors. Proceedings of the Environmental Sensitivities Workshop. Chronic Dis Canada. January 1991.

Appendix D

Position Statement of the California Medical Association

Clinical Ecology—A Critical Appraisal

In 1981 the California Medical Association (CMA) adopted the position that clinical ecology does not constitute a valid medical discipline and that scientific and clinical evidence to support the diagnosis of "environmental illness" and "cerebral allergy" or the concept of massive environmental allergy is lacking. As a result of requests from clinical ecologists for an opportunity to present to CMA evidence justifying their diagnostic and treatment methods, the chair of the CMA Scientific Board, Allen W. Mathies Jr., M.D., appointed a task force in 1984 to review clinical ecology. The task force conducted an extensive literature review and held a hearing.

Clinical ecology is based on two main hypotheses: First, that the total load of low-dose environmental stressors is important in the induction of illness; and, second, that changes in the frequency of and intervals between exposures to specific substances can mask the clinical manifestations of or alter the degree of sensitivity to those substances. Treatment methods used by clinical ecologists include avoidance,

From California Medical Association Scientific Board Task Force on Clinical Ecology: Clinical ecology—A critical appraisal. Western Journal of Medicine 144:239–245, 1986. Reprinted with permission.

symptom-neutralizing doses of diluted extract of the offending agents, rotation diets, and an ecologically sound workplace and home.

The task force recognizes that certain environmental chemicals and allergens produce well-defined syndromes in humans and that some patients suffer from illnesses that are not readily diagnosed and for which only supportive therapy exists. The conclusions of the task force are:

- There is no convincing evidence that supports the hypotheses on which clinical ecology is based.

- Clinical ecologists have not identified specific, recognizable diseases caused by exposure to low-level environmental stressors.

- Methods to diagnose and treat such undefined conditions have not been shown to be effective.

- The practice of clinical ecology can be considered experimental only when its practitioners adhere to scientifically sound research protocols and inform their patients about the experimental nature of their practice.

The practice of clinical ecology has been proposed as an alternative approach to the practice of environmental medicine. Practitioners of clinical ecology maintain that a broad range of common physical and psychological disorders can be triggered in susceptible persons by ongoing low-level exposure to foods, environmental chemicals, and natural inhalants. Because the medical community has been reluctant to accept clinical ecology concepts, many practitioners of clinical ecology are redesignating their treatment practices "allergy and environmental medicine."

This paper is the result of deliberations by the California Medical Association (CMA) Scientific Board's Task Force to Evaluate Clinical Ecology. In 1981 the CMA Scientific Board reviewed clinical ecology in cooperation with the CMA Scientific Advisory Panels on Allergy, Internal Medicine, Pediatrics and Preventive Medicine and Public Health, and the Committee on Environmental Health. The conclusions of this review were:

- Clinical ecology does not constitute a valid medical discipline.

• Scientific and clinical evidence to support the diagnosis of "environmental illness" and "cerebral allergy" or the concept of massive environmental allergy is lacking.

Because of repeated requests from some clinical ecologists for an opportunity to present to CMA evidence justifying their diagnostic and treatment methods, the chair of the Scientific Board, Allen W. Mathies Jr., M.D., appointed a task force in August 1984. The charge to the task force was to review pertinent material, to conduct a hearing at which clinical ecology proponents could present their views, and to formulate recommendations to the CMA. The task force did not address any political or economic issues but strictly limited itself to a scientific evaluation of the evidence. The three main questions the task force addressed were as follows:

1. Are there certain symptoms or signs that would allow physicians to identify specific diseases or syndromes induced by low-level environmental exposure as defined by clinical ecologists?

2. Do reliable tests exist that provide objective evidence of such diagnoses?

3. Are there proved therapies that are beneficial for patients who have been identified as having symptoms related to environmental exposure?

These questions were addressed by a review of available literature and at a hearing where practitioners of clinical ecology and others presented additional evidence. Before discussing the methodology, results, and conclusions of our appraisal, a brief overview of the basic tenets composing current clinical ecology practice is in order.

Overview of Clinical Ecology

Clinical ecology is based on two main hypotheses. First, the total load of low-dose environmental stressors is important in the induction of illness; and, second, changes in the frequency, intensity of, and intervals between exposure to a specific substance can mask the clinical manifestations of or alter the degree of sensitivity to that substance. Clinical ecologists focus on psychophysiological, psychiatric, and central nervous system syndromes. They believe that these are the results rather than the causes or correlates of sensitivities to environmental agents. Great emphasis is placed on the role of environmental chemicals and foods. The most common triggers of chronic ecologic illness are considered to be frequently ingested or inhaled substances including foods and indoor as well as outdoor air pollutants. Patients frequently are debilitated by their chronic symptoms.

Every system of the body may be affected. Symptoms and signs include depression, irritability, mood swings, inability to concentrate or think clearly, poor memory, fatigue or drowsiness; diarrhea, constipation, cramps, gas pain or bloating; sneezing, nasal congestion, runny nose, asthma, itching eyes and nose, eczema and skin rashes; and a diverse array of other symptoms such as headache, muscle and joint pain, swelling of various parts of the body, urinary frequency or pain, pounding heart, dark circles under the eyes, and cold or tingling extremities.

Potential stressors in the workplace, home, and external environment include practically everything that modern men and women come into contact with or use. Some of those identified are polluted urban air, diesel exhaust, tobacco smoke, fresh paint or tar, organic solvents and pesticides, new soft plastics, newspaper print, perfumes and colognes, unvented gas appliances, new building material and poorly ventilated new buildings, permanent press and synthetic fabrics, household cleaners, rubbing alcohol, felt-tip pens, cedar-lined closets, and tap water. Low doses of substances that alone might be benign may interact additively or synergistically on some common pathways in the body to produce illness. The greatest response to many stressors usually is evoked by the initial exposure after sensitization has been established. If exposure is frequent, however, the body may adapt by progressively dampening its acute response—but low-grade problems persist and are not easily recognized.

In contrast to allergic disorders, which are frequently IgE related and manifest themselves in the skin or in the respiratory system, environmental illnesses may be related to IgE and immune complexes— or other still unknown mechanisms—and may involve all bodily systems. The diagnosis of environmental illness is made by a detailed clinical, dietary, and environmental history. Suggestive laboratory evidence includes altered levels of T- and B-cell subsets. A patient's response is tested further by clinical avoidance and challenge tests, by serial dilution titration methods using skin tests, by provocation-neutralization tests, and by the cytotoxic test.

The endpoint dilution for a particular stressor is determined with the serial dilution titration method. Optimal dose treatment is then instituted with some fraction or multiple of values of the 0.01 ml endpoint dose with the goal to find the dose that will induce symptom relief for as long as possible between injections. In the provocation-neutralization test, a suspected offending substance is diluted and administered either intradermally or sublingually. The neutralizing dose is the concentration that relieves a patient's symptoms while a higher or lower dose will provoke symptoms. The cytotoxic blood test is based on the assumption that extracts of chemicals and foods to which the patient is sensitive will induce visible damage to the patient's platelets or leukocytes. The mainstays of treatment are avoidance or elimination of stressors in the diet or the environment, rotation diets, optimal dose intradermal treatment, neutralization treatment, and an ecologically sound workplace and home. Environmental control units play a prominent diagnostic and treatment role in some centers.

Methodology

Members of the task force were chosen for their expertise in internal medicine, toxicology, epidemiology, occupational medicine, allergy, immunology, pathology, neurology, and psychiatry. By necessity, the task force concentrated primarily on a thorough and critical review of the pertinent literature. Many references were provided by the petitioners. In addition, an independent search of the literature was conducted and articles were solicited from the American Academy of Environmental Medicine (formerly the Society for Clinical Ecology), the American Academy of Otolaryngic Allergy and the Pan-American Allergy Society. Key articles and books were reviewed by all members of the task force. Other articles requiring specific expertise were reviewed by individual members who then presented their findings to the group.

The task force agreed to accept certain criteria to make the literature review process as objective as possible. These criteria have been published,[1-3] but will be briefly summarized.

To assess *causation* of environmental illness, the following questions were raised:

1. Is there evidence from either experimental studies in humans (such as randomized controlled trials) or epidemiologic studies (such as cohort or case-control studies)?

2. Is the association strong?

3. Is the association consistent from study to study?

4. Is the temporal relationship correct?

5. Is there a dose-response relationship?

6. Does the association make epidemiologic sense?

7. Does the association make biologic sense?

8. Is the association specific?

9. Is the association consistent with a previously proved causal association?

To assess *prognosis* the following questions were asked:

1. Was an inception cohort assembled?

   a. Were patients identified at an early and uniform point in the course of their disease?

   b. Were the diagnostic criteria, disease, severity, co-morbidity, and demographic details for inclusion clearly specified?

2. Was a referral pattern described?

3. Was complete follow-up achieved?

4. Were objective outcome criteria developed and used?

5. Was outcome assessment blind?

6. Was adjustment for extraneous prognostic factors carried out?

Diagnostic tests were subjected to the following questions:

1. Was there an independent, "blind" comparison with a "gold standard" of diagnosis?

2. Was the setting for the study and the filter through which study patients passed adequately described?

3. Did the sample include an appropriate spectrum of mild and severe, treated and untreated patients, plus persons with different but commonly confused disorders?

4. Were the methods for carrying out the tests described in sufficient detail to permit their exact replication?

5. Was the reproducibility of the test result (precision) and its interpretation (observer variation) determined?

6. Was the term "normal" defined sensibly? (Gaussian; percentile; risk factor; culturally desirable, diagnostic, or therapeutic?)

7. If the test was advocated as part of a cluster or sequence of tests, was its contribution to the overall validity of the cluster or sequence determined?

8. Was the "utility" of the test determined? (Were patients really better off for it?)

Articles dealing with *therapy* were evaluated by asking the following questions:

1. Was the assignment of patients to treatments really random?
   a. Was similarity between groups documented?
   b. Was prognostic stratification used in allocation?
2. Were all clinically relevant outcomes reported?
   a. Were mortality and morbidity reported?
   b. Were deaths from all causes reported?
   c. Were quality of life assessments conducted?
   d. Was outcome assessment blind?
3. Were both statistical and clinical significance considered?
   a. If statistically significant, was the difference clinically important?
   b. Was the study population large enough to show a clinically important difference if it should occur?
4. Were all patients who entered the study accounted for at its conclusion? (Were dropouts, withdrawals, noncompliers, and those who crossed over handled appropriately in the analysis?)

A significant portion of the literature that was made available to the task force consisted of individual case reports, testimonials, and newspaper articles. While all materials were thoroughly reviewed, only publications that satisfied at least some of our review criteria were seriously considered.

Hearing

A hearing was conducted by the task force on April 30, 1985. Presenters were selected by the petitioners and the task force. Each presenter was given equal time. The presenters were John Boyles, M.D., President-Elect, American Academy of Otolaryngic Allergy; Jonathan Brostoff, M.D., Department of Immunology, Middlesex Hospital Medical School, London; Joel Bottler, Ph.D., Professor, Graduate Psychology Department, North Texas State University; Ronald Finn, M.D., Royal Liverpool Hospital, Liverpool, England; George R. Fricke, M.D., Allergist, Sacramento, California; Don L. Jewett, M.D., Associate Professor, Department of Orthopedics, University of California-San Francisco; Hal Levin, Professor, School of Architecture, University of California-Berkeley; William Rea, M.D., Clinical Associate Professor, University of Texas Southwestern Medical School, Dallas, Texas; and James C. Whittington, M.D., President-Elect, American Academy of Environmental Medicine, Fort Worth, Texas. The hearing was public and a number of interested persons attended. Because the purpose of the hearing was to gather additional information and to clarify certain unresolved questions, discussion was limited to presenters and task force members.

Some presentations were testimonials and others addressed known environmental pollutants and well-established disease entities not relevant to the charge of the task force. Still others provided some new data, but without the benefit of a detailed analysis of the study design, no judgment can be made at this time. Presenters were invited to send additional written information to the task force after the hearing and several did so.

Discussion of Published and Unpublished Papers

The task force was not charged with and did not conduct an extensive review of established allergic disorders and known or suspected environmental pollutants. Because material addressing these issues was submitted, we did review it but did not include it in our assessment. The task force also reviewed numerous publications that, by their nature, do not lend themselves for critical analysis or do not contain information that would be helpful to illuminate or answer the questions raised. These publications ... include books, editorials, position and policy statements, newspaper articles, symptom lists, letters, medical reports, case reports, course outlines, papers or presentations dealing with known or suspected pollutants, political statements, publications dealing with issues of medical quality assurance and legal aspects, review articles, research proposals, instruction papers, manuals, and books and articles of unknown source.

The following section will discuss papers reviewed by the task force which either appeared relevant to our inquiry, or which the petitioners offered as evidence documenting the efficacy of diagnostic and treatment methods in clinical ecology, or which satisfied at least some of our review criteria.

Three papers by Miller were reviewed. The first, a double-blind study of food extract injection therapy,[4] was found to contain statistically inappropriate data analysis. The second paper by the same author[5] is a discussion of the previous paper using the same patient population. Miller's third paper, "Treatment of Active Herpes Virus Infections with Influenza Virus Vaccine,"[6] was not a blinded study nor were the patients randomly assigned. A study by Burr and Merrett,[7] which represents a community survey of food intolerance in Great Britain, reported no association between food intolerance and allergic histories and also found that plasma IgE was lower in women with food intolerance. The study by Gardner and coworkers[8] investigating the role of plant and animal phenols in food allergy simply reported observations of 100 patients without random assignment.

The Society for Clinical Ecology, in a statement submitted to the California Board of Medical Quality Assurance,[9] cited the three papers reviewed below as best demonstrating the validity of the basic hypotheses of clinical ecology.

McGovern and associates[10] published a paper on food and chemical sensitivity describing six allergic patients and six normal controls. There was no definition of the disease entity being diagnosed or treated. Before challenge testing, the normal subjects showed no blood abnormalities, but the patients showed a mean of 3.7 abnormalities among the 15 immunopharmacologic components measured in their plasma. The most common abnormalities noted were depressed levels of epinephrine and IgE and elevated levels of CH-100. That allergic subjects are different immunologically from nonallergic subjects is not surprising. This study did not address the issue of provocation-neutralization or the efficacy of any treatment. Patients were not differentiated from controls and no criteria were given for patient selection and the filtering process. Similar problems were encountered in the study by Rea.

Rea and associates[11] addressed the issue of subcutaneous injection of food extracts in a neutralizing dose to reduce symptoms related to food allergies. From their general patient population the authors selected a subgroup of persons who could be "neutralized." Diagnostic criteria were not specified. Subjects apparently had experienced one of multiple symptoms, many vague and not objectively measurable, after oral food challenge. Subjects, testing technicians, and observers were ignorant of the content of each injection until after the response was judged to be positive or negative. The technician knew that one dose was neutralizing and two were placebos. Thus, if the first dose was neutralizing, the technician would know that the next two were placebos, which could influence the judgment of the observing technician. If the injections were truly random, the technician would know what the dose was in 27 cases and not know in 37 cases. Because the technician would know nearly half the time what was being administered, this study cannot be considered a truly blind evaluation. Further, even if this study had no methodological flaws, it is not justifiable to assume that results obtained in a highly selected group of patients are applicable to the general clinical ecology patient population. A study by Boris and coworkers[12] dealt with patients with asthma. The patients were their own controls, with pulmonary function measured in response to an inhalation challenge with antigen before and after injection of the "neutralizing" dose or placebo. The relevance of this study to populations without history of asthma must be seriously questioned. It is unlikely to be relevant to other populations simply defined as "chemically sensitized."

A study by Miller[13] presented information on eight cases treated by alternating neutralizing doses with doses of placebo. The order of the neutralizing dose and placebo was started randomly but then alternated. Presumably the patients did not know what they were receiving and the physician judging the complaints did not know what the patients were receiving. In general, there was a correlation between decreased symptoms and the use of a neutralizing dose. Sometimes administration of the placebo caused the symptoms to return and in three cases it did not. In these three cases in which symptoms did not return while the patient received a placebo, this was referred to as a "holdover" phenomenon. In other words, no matter what the result in these three persons, it could be explained. These eight cases were presented as eight cases in succession. If these were eight cases in succession, if the patients did not know what they were receiving and if the person who judged the symptoms was blinded, this paper does provide some evidence that neutralizing doses can be useful in relieving some symptoms. Nevertheless, since the interpretation by the investigator indicates that regardless of outcome, patients who received the neutralizing dose would improve, this study cannot be accepted as sound evidence.

In a 1983 study conducted by D. L. Jewett, M.D., and M. R. Greenberg, M.D., Department of Orthopedic Surgery, University of California, San Francisco, and presented at the April 30 hearing, 18 subjects in 8 different clinical ecology offices were tested under double-blind conditions to determine whether or not food extracts below a so-called neutralizing dose would provoke symptoms. Patients were selected by their treating physicians. Only subjects were entered who, under unblinded conditions, had been shown to have symptoms reliably provoked by injection of food extracts and relieved by neutralizing doses—but who had shown no reaction to injections of saline. In the experimental, double-blinded situation, the ratio of symptoms to injections was identical for both the active and the control injections (27 percent and 26 percent, respectively). Therefore, in this study, symptom provocation by intradermal testing of food extracts represents a placebo response.

A.I. Terr, M.D., evaluated 50 patients who had been previously diagnosed by 16 different clinical ecologists as having environmental illness.[14] In 41 patients the result of provocation-neutralization testing was used by clinical ecologists to support their diagnosis. All 50 patients received some form of clinical ecologic treatment. Clinical histories and offending chemicals were so heterogeneous that no patterns of symptomatology emerged to define a disease, syndrome, or nosologic entity. In only 2 of the 50 patients was there diminution in number and severity of symptoms as reported by the patient. In spite of treatment, 26 reported no change in their symptoms while 22 worsened. This group of patients does not represent a random sample but the observations suggest that a number of patients with environmental illnesses diagnosed by clinical ecologists do not benefit or are even made worse while under treatment by a clinical ecologist.

Conclusions

The task force collected material as for any subject review and included all information supplied by individual clinical ecologists and by their professional organizations. There was extensive description of the basic hypotheses of clinical ecology, and an ample and varied collection of anecdotal reports and individual patient testimonials. In contrast, there was a surprising paucity of published studies to prove or disprove clinical ecology hypotheses. Critical analyses of patients and cohorts, detailed data collection, validation and confirming laboratory assays were not provided.

No convincing evidence was found that patients treated by clinical ecologists have unique, recognizable syndromes, that the diagnostic tests employed are efficacious and reliable or that the treatments used are effective. Even though clinical ecology has existed for approximately 50 years, only a few studies have been conducted that are scientifically sound. Most have such serious methodological flaws as to make their conclusions unacceptable. Those few studies that used scientifically sound methods have provided evidence that the effectiveness of certain treatment methods used by clinical ecologists is based principally on placebo response.

Undoubtedly, some patients suffer from illnesses that cannot be readily diagnosed and for which only supportive treatments exist. It may even be true that some or all of the hypotheses and treatments proposed by clinical ecologists are valid but we found no evidence to support them. These hypotheses and treatments should be subjected to modern, scientific methods of evaluation. We think that this can be done provided genuine interest exists.

The task force is concerned that unproved diagnostic tests are being widely used by clinical ecologists in what may be incorrect or inappropriate applications. Decisions made on the basis of these tests can lead to misdiagnosis, resulting in patients being denied other supportive treatments and becoming psychologically dependent, believing themselves seriously and chronically impaired. This possibility underscores the need for more adequate scientific studies to prove or disprove the value of clinical ecology tests and treatments. To consider the current practice of clinical ecology experimental is misleading, however. It can only be considered experimental when its practitioners adhere to scientifically sound research protocols and inform their patients about the investigative nature of their practice.

Appendix:
Scientific Board Task Force on Clinical Ecology

W. C. Wiederholt, M.D. (Chair), Professor of Neurosciences, University of California-San Diego; Charles Becker, M.D., Chief, Division of Occupational Medicine, San Francisco General Hospital; Carroll Brodsky, M.D., Professor of Psychiatry, Langley Porter Psychiatric Institute, San Francisco, California; Gideon Letz, M.D., Chief, Hazard Evaluation System and Information Service, State Department of Health Services; Michael Miller, M.D., Chair, Department of Pediatrics, University of California-Davis; John Peters, M.D., Director, Division of Occupational Health, University of Southern California; Edward Smuckler, M.D., Chief, Department of Pathology, University of California-San Francisco; Stephen Wasserman, M.D., Professor of Medicine, University of California-San Diego; Antony Gualtieri, M.D., Consultant, Chief Medical Consultant, Board of Medical Quality Assurance, Sacramento, California; and Linda Ramsey, Director, Division of Scientific and Educational Activities, California Medical Association.

References

1. How to read clinical journals: II. To learn about a diagnostic test. Can Med Assoc J 124:869–872, 1981.
2. How to read clinical journals: III. To determine etiology or causation. Can Medical Assoc J 124:985–990, 1981.
3. How to read clinical journals: IV. To distinguish useful from useless or even harmful therapy. Can Med Assoc J 124:1156–1162, 1981.
4. Miller J. A double-blind study of food extract injection therapy: A preliminary report. Ann Allergy 38:185–191, 1977.
5. Miller J. The optimal dose method of food allergy management. J Cont Educ ORL Allergy 40:37–50, 1978.
6. Miller J. Treatment of active herpes virus infections with influenza virus vaccine. Ann Allergy 42:295–305, 1979.
7. Burr ML, Merrett TG. Food intolerance: A community survey. Br Nutr 42:217–219, 1983.
8. Gardner R, McGovern J, Brenneman L. The Role of Plant and Animal Phenyl in Food Allergy. Presented at 37th Annual Congress American College of Allergy. Washington, D.C., Apr. 1981.
9. The Society for Clinical Ecology. A plea for thoughtful consideration. Submitted to the Board of Medical Quality Assurance. San Francisco, 1985.
10. McGovern J, Lazaroni J, Hicks M, and others. Food and chemical sensitivity: Clinical and immunologic correlates. Arch Otolaryngol 109:292–297, 1983.

11. Rea J, Podell R, Williams M, and others. Elimination of oral food challenge reaction by injection of food extracts. Arch Otolaryngol 110:248–252, 1984.
12. Boris M, Weindorf S, Corriel RN, and others. Allergic Asthma Due to Animal Allergens: Protection from Bronchial Provocation by Neutralizing Doses of Allergen. Department of Pediatrics, North Shore University Hospital, Manhasset, N.Y. (unpublished paper)
13. Miller J. Neutralization therapy update. In Spencer JT, editor. Allergy: Immunologic and Management Considerations. Miami: Meded Publishers 1982:43–54.
14. Terr AI. Environmental illness: A clinical review of fifty cases. Arch Intern Med 146:145–149, 1986.

An appendix listing 125 additional source documents is not reproduced in this book.

Appendix E

Daubert v. *Merrell Dow*
The Supreme Court's Ruling
on Expert Testimony

In this case we are called upon to determine the standard for admitting expert scientific testimony in a federal trial.

Petitioners Jason Daubert and Eric Schuller are minor children born with serious birth defects. They and their parents sued respondent in California state court, alleging that the birth defects had been caused by the mothers' ingestion of Bendectin, a prescription antinausea drug marketed by respondent. . . .

After extensive discovery, respondent [the company] moved for summary judgment, contending that Bendectin does not cause birth defects in humans and that petitioners would be unable to come forward with any admissible evidence that it does. In support of its motion, respondent submitted an affidavit of Steven H. Lamm, physician and epidemiologist, who is a well-credentialed expert on the risks from exposure to various chemical substances. Doctor Lamm stated that he had reviewed all the literature on Bendectin and human birth defects—more than 30 published studies involving over 130,000 patients. No study had found Bendectin to be a human teratogen (i.e., a substance capable of causing malformations in fetuses). On the basis of this review,

This appendix contains the significant language of the U.S. Supreme Court's ruling on June 23, 1993, in the case of *William Daubert, et ux., etc., et al., Petitioners,* v. *Merrell Dow Pharmaceuticals, Inc.* The legal citations are not included.

Doctor Lamm concluded that maternal use of Bendectin during the first trimester of pregnancy has not been shown to be a risk factor for human birth defects.

Petitioners did not (and do not) contest this characterization of the published record regarding Bendectin. Instead, they responded to respondent's motion with the testimony of eight experts of their own, each of whom also possessed impressive credentials. These experts had concluded that Bendectin can cause birth defects. Their conclusions were based upon "in vitro" (test tube) and "in vivo" (live) animal studies that found a link between Bendectin and malformations; pharmacological studies of the chemical structure of Bendectin that purported to show similarities between the structure of the drug and that of other substances known to cause birth defects; and the "reanalysis" of previously published epidemiological (human statistical) studies.

The District Court granted respondent's motion for summary judgment. The court stated that scientific evidence is admissible only if the principle upon which it is based is "sufficiently established to have general acceptance in the field to which it belongs." The court concluded that petitioners' evidence did not meet this standard. Given the vast body of epidemiological data concerning Bendectin, the court held, expert opinion which is not based on epidemiological evidence is not admissible to establish causation. Thus, the animal-cell studies, live-animal studies, and chemical structure analyses on which petitioners had relied could not raise by themselves a reasonably disputable jury issue regarding causation. Petitioners' epidemiological analyses, based as they were on recalculations of data in previously published studies that had found no causal link between the drug and birth defects, were ruled to be inadmissible because they had not been published or subjected to peer review.

The United States Court of Appeals for the Ninth Circuit affirmed. Citing *Frye* v. *United States* (1923), the court stated that expert opinion based on a scientific technique is inadmissible unless the technique is "generally accepted" as reliable in the relevant scientific community. The court declared that expert opinion based on a methodology that diverges "significantly from the procedures accepted by recognized authorities in the field . . . cannot be shown to be 'generally accepted as a reliable technique.'"

The court emphasized that other Courts of Appeals considering the risks of Bendectin had refused to admit reanalyses of epidemiological studies that had been neither published nor subjected to peer review. Those courts had found unpublished reanalyses "particularly problematic in light of the massive weight of the original published studies supporting [respondent's] position, all of which had undergone full scrutiny from the scientific community." Contending that reanalysis is generally accepted by the scientific community only when it is subjected to verification and scrutiny by others in the field, the Court of Appeals rejected petitioners' reanalyses as "unpublished, not subjected to the normal peer review process and generated solely for use in litigation." The court concluded that petitioners' evidence provided an insufficient foundation to allow admission of expert testimony that Bendectin caused their injuries and, accordingly, that petitioners could not satisfy their burden of proving causation at trial.

We granted certiorari, in light of sharp divisions among the courts regarding the proper standard for the admission of expert testimony. [*Authors' note*: Certiorari is a writ from a higher court to a lower one requesting a transcript of the proceedings of a case for review.]

II A

In the 70 years since its formulation in the *Frye* case, the "general acceptance" test has been the dominant standard for determining the admissibility of novel scientific evidence at trial. Although under increasing attack of late, the rule continues to be followed by a majority of courts, including the Ninth Circuit.

The *Frye* test has its origin in a short and citation-free 1923 decision concerning the admissibility of evidence derived from a systolic blood pressure deception test, a crude precursor to the polygraph machine. In what has become a famous (perhaps infamous) passage, the then Court of Appeals for the District of Columbia described the device and its operation and declared:

> Just when a scientific principle or discovery crosses the line between the experimental and demonstrable stages is difficult to define. Somewhere in this twilight zone the evidential force of the principle must be recognized, and while courts will go a long

way in admitting expert testimony deduced from a well recognized scientific principle or discovery, *the thing from which the deduction is made must be sufficiently established to have gained general acceptance in the particular field in which it belongs* [emphasis added].

Because the deception test had "not yet gained such standing and scientific recognition among physiological and psychological authorities as would justify the courts in admitting expert testimony deduced from the discovery, development, and experiments thus far made," evidence of its results was ruled inadmissible.

The merits of the *Frye* test have been much debated, and scholarship on its proper scope and application is legion. Petitioners' primary attack, however, is not on the content but on the continuing authority of the rule. They contend that the *Frye* test was superseded by the adoption of the Federal Rules of Evidence. We agree.

We interpret the legislatively enacted Federal Rules of Evidence as we would any statute. Rule 402 provides the baseline:

All relevant evidence is admissible, except as otherwise provided by the Constitution of the United States, by Act of Congress, by these rules, or by other rules prescribed by the Supreme Court pursuant to statutory authority. Evidence which is not relevant is not admissible.

"Relevant evidence" is defined as that which has "any tendency to make the existence of any fact that is of consequence to the determination of the action more probable or less probable than it would be without the evidence." (Rule 401.) The Rule's basic standard of relevance thus is a liberal one.

Frye, of course, predated the Rules by half a century. In *United States* v. *Abel,* we considered the pertinence of background common law in interpreting the Rules of Evidence. We noted that the Rules occupy the field, but, quoting Professor Cleary, the Reporter explained that the common law nevertheless could serve as an aid to their application:

In principle, under the Federal Rules no common law of evidence remains. All relevant evidence is admissible, except as otherwise provided. In reality, of course, the body of common law knowledge continues to exist, though in the somewhat altered form of a source of guidance in the exercise of delegated powers.

We found the common-law precept at issue in the *Abel* case entirely consistent with Rule 402's general requirement of admissibility, and considered it unlikely that the drafters had intended to change the rule. In *Bourjaily* v. *United States,* on the other hand, the Court was unable to find a particular common-law doctrine in the Rules, and so held it superseded.

Here there is a specific rule that speaks to the contested issue. Rule 702, governing expert testimony, provides:

> If scientific, technical, or other specialized knowledge will assist the trier of fact to understand the evidence or to determine a fact in issue, a witness qualified as an expert by knowledge, skill, experience, training, or education, may testify thereto in the form of an opinion or otherwise.

Nothing in the text of this Rule establishes "general acceptance" as an absolute prerequisite to admissibility. Nor does respondent present any clear indication that Rule 702 or the Rules as a whole were intended to incorporate a "general acceptance" standard. The drafting history makes no mention of *Frye,* and a rigid "general acceptance" requirement would be at odds with the "liberal thrust" of the Federal Rules and their "general approach of relaxing the traditional barriers to 'opinion' testimony." ("The Rules were designed to depend primarily upon lawyer-adversaries and sensible triers of fact to evaluate conflicts.") Given the Rules' permissive backdrop and their inclusion of a specific rule on expert testimony that does not mention "general acceptance," the assertion that the Rules somehow assimilated *Frye* is unconvincing. *Frye* made 'general acceptance' the exclusive test for admitting expert scientific testimony. That austere standard, absent from and incompatible with the Federal Rules of Evidence, should not be applied in federal trials.

II B

That the *Frye* test was displaced by the Rules of Evidence does not mean, however, that the Rules themselves place no limits on the admissibility of purportedly scientific evidence. Nor is the trial judge disabled from screening such evidence. To the contrary, under the Rules the trial judge must ensure that any and all scientific testimony or evidence admitted is not only relevant, but reliable.

The primary locus of this obligation is Rule 702, which clearly contemplates some degree of regulation of the subjects and theories about which an expert may testify. "If scientific, technical, or other specialized knowledge will assist the trier of fact to understand the evidence or to determine a fact in issue" an expert "may testify thereto." The subject of an expert's testimony must be "scientific . . . knowledge." The adjective "scientific" implies a grounding in the methods and procedures of science. Similarly, the word "knowledge" connotes more than subjective belief or unsupported speculation. The term "applies to any body of known facts or to any body of ideas inferred from such facts or accepted as truths on good grounds." Of course, it would be unreasonable to conclude that the subject of scientific testimony must be "known" to a certainty; arguably, there are no certainties in science. [Briefs submitted in this case by scientific organizations state] "Indeed, scientists do not assert that they know what is immutably 'true'—they are committed to searching for new, temporary theories to explain, as best they can, phenomena," [and] "Science is not an encyclopedic body of knowledge about the universe. Instead, it represents a *process* for proposing and refining theoretical explanations about the world that are subject to further testing and refinement." But, in order to qualify as "scientific knowledge," an inference or assertion must be derived by the scientific method. Proposed testimony must be supported by appropriate validation—i.e., "good grounds," based on what is known. In short, the requirement that an expert's testimony pertain to "scientific knowledge" establishes a standard of evidentiary reliability.

Rule 702 further requires that the evidence or testimony "assist the trier of fact to understand the evidence or to determine a fact in issue." This condition goes primarily to relevance. "Expert testimony which does not relate to any issue in the case is not relevant and, ergo, nonhelpful." ("An additional consideration under Rule 702—and another aspect of relevancy—is whether expert testimony proffered in the case is sufficiently tied to the facts of the case that it will aid the jury in resolving a factual dispute.") The consideration has been aptly described by Judge Becker as one of "fit." "Fit" is not always obvious, and scientific validity for one purpose is not necessarily scientific validity for other, unrelated purposes. The study of the phases of the moon, for example, may provide valid scientific "knowledge" about whether a certain night was dark, and if darkness is a fact in issue, the knowledge will assist the trier of fact. However (absent creditable grounds supporting such a link), evidence that the moon was full on a certain night will not assist the trier of fact in determining whether an individual was unusually likely to have behaved irrationally on that night. Rule 702's "helpfulness" standard requires a valid scientific connection to the pertinent inquiry as a precondition to admissibility.

That these requirements are embodied in Rule 702 is not surprising. Unlike an ordinary witness (see Rule 701), an expert is permitted wide latitude to offer opinions, including those that are not based on firsthand knowledge or observation. (See Rules 702 and 703.) Presumably, this relaxation of the usual requirement of firsthand knowledge—a rule which represents "a 'most pervasive manifestation' of the common law insistence upon 'the most reliable sources of information' "—is premised on an assumption that the expert's opinion will have a reliable basis in the knowledge and experience of his discipline.

II C

Faced with a proffer of expert scientific testimony, then, the trial judge must determine at the outset, pursuant to Rule 104(a), whether the expert is proposing to testify to (1) scientific knowledge that (2) will assist the trier of fact to understand or determine a fact in issue. This entails a preliminary assessment of whether the reasoning or methodology underlying the testimony is scientifically valid and of whether that reasoning or methodology properly can be applied to the facts in issue. We are confident that federal judges possess the capacity to undertake this review. Many factors will bear on the inquiry, and we do not presume to set out a definitive checklist or test. But some general observations are appropriate.

Ordinarily, a key question to be answered in determining whether a theory or technique is scientific knowledge that will assist the trier of fact will be whether it can be (and has been) tested. "Scientific methodology today is based on generating hypotheses and testing them to see if they can be falsified; indeed, this methodology is what distinguishes science from other fields of human inquiry." [Scientific authorities have noted that] "the statements constituting a scientific explanation must be capable of empirical test" [and] "the criterion of the scientific status of a theory is its falsifiability, or refutability, or testability."

Another pertinent consideration is whether the theory or technique has been subjected to peer review and publication. Publication (which is but one element of peer review) is not a *sine qua non* of admissibility; it does not necessarily correlate with reliability, and in some instances well-grounded but innovative theories will not have been published. Some propositions, moreover, are too particular, too new, or of too limited interest to be published. But submission to the scrutiny of the scientific community is a component of "good science," in part because it increases the likelihood that substantive flaws in methodology will be detected. The fact of publication (or lack thereof) in a peer-reviewed journal thus will be a relevant, though not dispositive, consideration in assessing the scientific validity of a particular technique or methodology on which an opinion is premised.

Additionally, in the case of a particular scientific technique, the court ordinarily should consider the known or potential rate of error and the existence and maintenance of standards controlling the technique's operation.

Finally, "general acceptance" can yet have a bearing on the inquiry. A "reliability assessment does not require, although it does permit, explicit identification of a relevant scientific community and an express determination of a particular degree of acceptance within that community." Widespread acceptance can be an important factor in ruling particular evidence admissible, and "a known technique that has been able to attract only minimal support within the community" may properly be viewed with skepticism.

The inquiry envisioned by Rule 702 is, we emphasize, a flexible one. Its overarching subject is the scientific validity—and thus the evidentiary relevance and reliability—of the principles that underlie a proposed submission. The focus, of course, must be solely on principles and methodology, not on the conclusions that they generate.

Throughout, a judge assessing a proffer of expert scientific testimony under Rule 702 should also be mindful of other applicable rules. Rule 703 provides that expert opinions based on otherwise inadmissible hearsay are to be admitted only if the facts or data are "of a type reasonably relied upon by experts in the particular field in forming opinions or inferences upon the subject." Rule 706 allows the court at its discretion to procure the assistance of an expert of its own choosing. Finally, Rule 403 permits the exclusion of relevant evidence "if its probative value is substantially outweighed by the danger of unfair prejudice, confusion of the issues, or misleading the jury. . ." Judge Weinstein has explained: "Expert evidence can be both powerful and quite misleading because of the difficulty in evaluating it. Because of this risk, the judge in weighing possible prejudice against probative force under Rule 403 of the present rules exercises more control over experts than over lay witnesses."

III

We conclude by briefly addressing what appear to be two underlying concerns of the parties and *amici* in this case. [*Authors' note*: An *amicus curiae* is an outside party who files a "friend of the court" legal brief.] Respondent expresses apprehension that abandonment of "general acceptance" as the exclusive requirement for admission will result in a "free-for-all" in which befuddled juries are confounded by absurd and irrational pseudoscientific assertions. In this regard respondent seems to us to be overly pessimistic about the capabilities of the jury, and of the adversary system generally. Vigorous cross-examination, presentation of contrary evidence, and careful instruction on the burden of proof are the traditional and appropriate means of attacking shaky but admissible evidence. Additionally, in the event the trial court concludes that the scintilla of evidence presented supporting a position is insufficient to allow a reasonable juror to conclude that the position more likely than not is true, the court remains free to direct a judgment and likewise to grant a summary judgment. These conventional devices, rather than wholesale exclusion under an uncompromising "general acceptance" test, are the appropriate standards where the basic scientific testimony meets the standards of Rule 702.

Petitioners and, to a greater extent, their *amici* exhibit a different concern. They suggest that recognition of a screening role for a judge that allows exclusion of "invalid" evidence will sanction a stifling and repressive medical orthodoxy and will be inimical to the search for truth. It is true that open debate is an essential part of both legal and scientific analyses. Yet there are important differences between the search for truth in the courtroom and the quest for truth in the laboratory. Scientific conclusions are subject to perpetual revision. Law, on the other hand, must resolve disputes finally and quickly. The scientific project is advanced by broad and wide-ranging consideration of a multitude of hypotheses, for those that are incorrect will eventually be shown to be so, and that in itself is an advance. Conjectures that are wrong are of little use, however, in the project of reaching a quick, final, and binding legal judgment—often of great consequence—about a particular set of events in the past. We recognize that in practice, a gatekeeping role for the judge, no matter how flexible, inevitably on occasion will prevent the jury from learning of authentic insights and innovations. That, nevertheless, is the balance that is struck by Rules of Evidence designed not for the exhaustive search for cosmic understanding but for the particularized resolution of legal disputes.

IV

To summarize: "general acceptance" is not a necessary precondition to the admissibility of scientific evidence under the Federal Rules of Evidence, but the Rules of Evidence—especially Rule 702—do assign to the trial judge the task of ensuring that an expert's testimony both rests on a reliable foundation and is relevant to the task at hand. Pertinent evidence based on scientifically valid principles will satisfy those demands.

The inquiries of the District Court and the Court of Appeals focused almost exclusively on "general acceptance," as gauged by publication and the decisions of other courts. Accordingly, the judgment of the Court of Appeals is vacated and the case is remanded for further proceedings consistent with this opinion.

It is so ordered.

Appendix F

Court Rulings
Unfavorable to MCS

Bahura et al. **v.** *S.E.W. Investors et al.* The trial court judge overturned four out of five jury verdicts favoring plaintiffs in a "sick building syndrome" action brought by Environmental Protection Agency workers at the Waterside Mall Office Complex. Plaintiffs claimed to have MCS toxic encephalopathy caused by building renovations. Dr. Iris Bell's testimony on the "limbic kindling" hypothesis was excluded as unreliable. [This theory is described in the Glossary.] The judge noted that she had acknowledged that this was not generally accepted in the fields of psychiatry or neurology, and that low-level exposure to everyday chemicals does not cause permanent injury. [No. 90-CA-10594, District of Columbia Superior Court, Nov. 29, 1995]

Benney **v.** *Shaw Industries, Inc.* The court excluded the opinion of Dr. Hildegarde Staninger that plaintiff's MCS was caused by carpeting and a "bug bomb" as his methodology was unreliable. The court also excluded as unreliable the testing of Dr. Alan Broughton's laboratory as not the type reasonably relied upon by experts in the field. [No. 93-685-CIT-T-21(A), Middle District, Florida, 1995]

Bloomquist **v.** *Wappello County et al.* The judge overturned a $1,000,000 verdict for two employees of a "sick building," ruling that plaintiffs' clinical ecology evidence was "unproven medical speculation which is

---

These summaries were prepared with help from Timothy E. Kapshandy, J.D., a partner in the law firm of Sidley & Austin (Chicago office). Mr. Kapshandy specializes in litigation involving scientific evidence, including the defense of claims from exposure to low levels of chemicals and other substances.

not accepted by mainstream medicine." [Mahaska City, Iowa, Dist. Ct. No. CL0174-0687 [Aug. 28, 1990] The Iowa Supreme Court later reversed the judge's ruling, holding that epidemiologic evidence was not required. [No. 419/90-1371, Iowa Sup. Ct., April 21, 1993]

Bradley v. *Brown.* Two federal courts excluded testimony of Drs. William Rea and Alfred Johnson. The trial court found their methodology anecdotal and speculative. Regarding the general concept of MCS, the court held that scientific knowledge about its etiology has not progressed from hypothesis to knowledge capable of assisting the jury. [No. CIV-H85-958, 1994 WL 199827, Northern District, Indiana, May 17, 1994, affirmed, No. 94-2467, 7th Circuit, Dec. 13, 1994]

Brandon v. *First Republicbank Group Medical Plan.* A federal judge ruled that the services of clinical ecologists Drs. William Rea and Alfred Johnson were not medically necessary and therefore not coverable under an employee welfare benefit plan. [No. CA-7-89-002, Northern District, Texas, Nov. 27, 1990]

Brown v. *Shalala.* An administrative law judge ruled that the plaintiff was not entitled to Social Security disability benefits because her diagnosis of environmental illness, using techniques such as sublingual testing, was not based on medically acceptable clinical and laboratory techniques. The ruling was upheld on appeal by both the federal court and the federal court of appeals. [15 F.3d 97, 8th Circuit, 1994]

Carlin v. *RFE Industries et al.* The judge excluded the testimony of Drs. James Miller and Michael B. Lax that plaintiff had MCS from exposure to solvents used in the manufacture of circuit boards. The court held that the diagnosis was not based on reliable methods and that the general validity and etiology of MCS had not been established. [No. 88-CV-842, Northern District, New York, Nov. 27, 1995]

Carroll v. *Litton Systems.* A federal judge excluded the lymphocyte testing and autoantibody testing of Dr. Alan Broughton as lacking a proper factual basis (i.e., no proper controls; alternative causes not excluded). [No. B-C-88-253, Western District, North Carolina, Oct. 29, 1990] The judge's ruling was reversed on other grounds. [No. 92-2219, 4th Circuit, Jan. 13, 1995]

Carroll v. *Marion County Board of Education.* A state jury sided with the defense in one of several cases brought by families who sued for students' alleged long-term exposure to pesticides. The judge precluded clinical ecologist Grace Ziem, M.D., from testifying that the plaintiff's son suffered from MCS. The judge said: (1) MCS did not pass the "good science" test, (2) the diagnosis of MCS had been almost universally rejected by the medical and scientific community, and (3) the methodology supporting MCS was "somewhat suspect." [No. 92-C-196, W. Va. Circuit, Marion Co., Div 1]

Cavallo v. Star Enterprise et al. Plaintiff claimed that she had chronic respiratory illnesses through exposure to aviation jet fuel (AvJet) while walking across a parking lot of a restaurant about 500 feet way from a distribution facility where a 34,000-gallon spill had taken place. The court concluded that the opinion of plaintiff's expert Dr. Joseph Bellanti were largely based on hypothesis and speculation. In granting summary judgment, the judge stated: "It may well be that AvJet spill forever 'sensitized' Ms. Cavallo to petroleum vapors and various household chemicals. But the published scientific literature and test results simply do not support that conclusion at any time." [No. 94-1499-A, Eastern District, Virginia, 1995]

Claar et al. v. Burlington Northern Railroad. Six plaintiffs were selected from 27 cases of railroad workers filed under the Federal Employees Liability Act (FELA) suffering from unspecified multiple chemical exposures. The U.S. District Court of Montana provided summary judgment for the railroad because plaintiffs' experts (Drs. Mark Hines and Richard Nelson) had failed to adequately explain the bases of their MCS diagnoses, specify which chemicals caused which injury, or rule out other possible causes. Plaintiffs argued that the court had erred in demanding that their experts demonstrate a causal connection between specific injuries and specific chemicals. The appellate court upheld the lower court, stating: "This argument misconceives both the standards for causation under FELA and its relationship to the Federal Rules of Evidence." [No. 92-35337, 92-35539, U.S. District Court, Montana; 9th Circuit Court of Appeals, July 14, 1994]

Conradt v. Mt. Carmel School Fireman's Fund Insurance Commission. The Wisconsin Court of Appeals upheld the Labor and Industry Review Commission's denial of plaintiff's claim (based on the opinion of Dr. Theron Randolph) that building materials at the school where she worked had caused her to develop MCS. The appeals court rejected claimant's contention that her treating physicians should be accorded more credibility than employer's experts. [No. 94-2842, Wisc. App. 2nd Dist., Sept. 27, 1995]

Frank v. New York. Plaintiffs alleged that exposure to pesticides and other chemicals had made them hypersensitive to normal levels of airborne chemicals and that their employer had failed to reasonably accommodate them as required under the Americans with Disabilities Act. The judge ruled that expert testimony about the cause of their alleged disability (MCS) would be too speculative to constitute "scientific knowledge." He also noted that the theory underlying MCS was "untested, speculative, and far from generally accepted in the medical or toxicological community." [No. 95-CV-399, U.S. District Court for the Northern District of New York, July 15, 1997]

Hundley* v. *Norfolk & Western Railway Co. The court excluded the opinions of Drs. Rea and Johnson that plaintiff's one-time exposure to herbicides at a railyard was the cause of his MCS. [No. 91C -6127, N.D. Ill., Jan, 31, 1996]

Kuehm* v. *Hearnen Air Conditioning. Plaintiff brought a "sick building syndrome" case alleging mite and fungal allergies due to a defective ventilation system. The trial court summarily dismissed the case, holding that her experts' speculation about conditions four years previous were not competent evidence. [No. A-4289-93T3, N.J. Super., App. Div., July 13, 1995]

La-Z-Boy Chair Co.* v. *Reed. The U.S. Court of Appeals for the Sixth Circuit affirmed the trial court's decision to bar the testimony of plaintiff's clinical ecologist, Fred Furr, M.D., that plaintiff was permanently disabled as a result of exposure to trichloromethane at work. The court held that such testimony was "only a theory which is not generally accepted by the medical profession." [No. 90-6013, 6th Circuit, June 28, 1991]

Donald and Susan Maxwell* v. *Sears, Roebuck & Co. et al. Despite testimony by Alan Lieberman, M.D., Albert Robbins, D.O., and Susan Franks, Ph.D., the judge concluded that "multiple chemical sensitivity is a theoretical hypothesis lacking sufficient scientific proof." Ruling that trial court must follow the "general acceptance" test set forth in *Frye* v. *United States*, the judge ordered all parties not to refer to MCS during the trial. [No. CA 94-0156, Fla. Circuit, Manatee Co., March 3, 1997]

Mullenax* v. *McRae's. The Mississippi Workers' Compensation Commission denied a claim that workplace exposure to solvents in art supplies had caused MCS. The Commission concluded that the unorthodox methodology of Dr. William Rea did not establish causal connection, and that even if they were to accept the theory that exposure to one chemical can cause multiple chemical sensitivities, other legitimate explanations were not excluded. [No. 87-13915-D-3130, Mississippi Workers' Compensation Commission, March 18, 1993]

Nethery* v. *Servicemaster Co. The trial court excluded the testimony of Drs. Thomas Glasgow and Alan Lieberman, holding that MCS is an "unproven theory." [No. 92-167(G)(L), Miss. Cir. Ct., Lee Co., Feb. 15, 1996]

Newman v. *Stringfellow*. The trial court ruled that plaintiff's immune assays, including calla and porphyrin antibody testing, performed by Dr. Bertram Carnow, were inadmissible because plaintiff failed to prove that the testing was "acceptable to at least a substantial minority of the relevant scientific community." [No. 165994, California Superior Court, Riverside County, Jan. 17, 1991]

In Re Paoli R. R. Yard PCB Litigation. The 3rd Circuit upheld the exclusion of the causation opinion of Dr. Janette Sherman for those plaintiffs on whom she did not perform the traditional clinical method (i.e., exam, history, etc.), but allowed it for those on whom she did. The court also excluded the immunological testing of Dr. Alan Broughton. [35F. 3rd 717, 3rd Circuit, 1994]

Phillips v. *Velsicol Chemical Corporation*. Plaintiff, a percussionist with the Hong Kong Philharmonic Orchestra, alleged MCS symptoms had resulted from a single pesticide exposure in a concert hall. The court excluded screening tests performed by Dr. Robert K. Simon of Accu-Chem Laboratories because they were scientifically unreliable and not trustworthy and failed to follow established protocol. Dr. William Rea's opinion regarding the harmful effects of chlordane on the plaintiff by "double-blind" tests were deemed irrelevant for lack of specifically identifying chlordane in the alleged incident in the concert hall. [No. 93-CV-140-J, District of Wyoming, Sept. 19, 1995]

Rea v. *Aetna Life Insurance Co.* A federal judge rejected plaintiff's attempt to bring a class action on behalf of clinical ecologists and their patients against Aetna and the American Academy of Allergy and Immunology, holding that plaintiffs failed to establish that clinical ecologists and their patients were a "recognizable and identifiable class." [No. 3-84-0219-H, Northern District, Texas, Feb. 25, 1985]

Rutigliano v. *Valley Business Forms*. The court excluded the opinion of Dr. Elaine Panitz that exposure to carbonless paper had made plaintiff sensitive to formaldehyde. The court noted that Panitz was basically a full-time witness who made her diagnosis after an initial visit, based on self-reported symptoms and history. The court also rejected her reliance on blood tests, done in Dr. Alan Broughton's lab, which she had accepted if supportive but dismissed if negative. [No. 90-1432, D.N.J. June 27, 1996]

Sanderson v. *International Flavors and Fragrances et al.* A federal judge summarily dismissed plaintiff's claim that exposure to perfumes and colognes over an eighteen-month period has caused her to develop MCS, toxic encephalopathy, and impairment of her sense of smell. The court held that the testimony of Drs. Nachman Brautbar, Gunnar Heuser, Richard Perillo, and Jack Thrasher were not sufficient to establish that her symptoms were caused by defendants' fragrance products. The judge also ruled that the plaintiff had failed to demonstrate that MCS is "good science." [No. CV-95-3387, C.D. Calif, Aug. 28, 1996]

Schickele v. Rhodes. The court excluded the testimony of clinical ecologist Alan Levin, M.D., who was planning to testify that plaintiff suffered from chemically induced immune system dysfunction syndrome as a result to exposure to hydrogen sulfide. [No. C 451843, Arizona Superior Court, Maricopa County, Aug. 1, 1986]

Sterling v. Velsicol Chemical Corp. The U.S. Court of Appeals for the 6th Circuit excluded from evidence the clinical ecology testimony of Dr. Alan Levin as generally unaccepted, based in part on the position papers of the American Academy of Allergy and Immunology and the California Medical Association, and reversed an award of damages for injuries to plaintiff's immune system. [855 F. 2d 1188, 6th Circuit, 1988]

Summers v. Missouri Pacific Railroad System. Railroad employees alleged they had developed chemical sensitivity and brain damage from short-term exposure to diesel exhaust fumes. The court excluded Dr. Alfred Johnson's testimony on the basis that the MCS hypothesis was unproven. The court also found his efforts to distinguish plaintiff's alleged "chemical sensitivity" from what was formerly called "multiple chemical sensitivity" unpersuasive. The testimony of psychologist Susan Franks, Ph.D., was also excluded. [No. 94-468-P, U.S. District Court, Eastern District, Oklahoma, Aug. 25, 1995]

Taylor v. Airport Transport and Warehouse Services, Ltd. A British court rejected the claim of plaintiff's clinical ecologist that her multiple chemical sensitivity was triggered by exposure to chemical fumes in a truck she was driving, holding that "her evidence was in many respects bizarre and unscientific . . . [and] unacceptable to the vast majority of doctors." [No. 90/NJ/5076, High Court of Justice, Queen's Bench Division, Oct. 24, 1991]

Valentine v. Pioneer Chlor Alkali. Plaintiffs alleged that they suffered neuropsychological injuries from chlorine gas. The court excluded the testimony of Drs. Kaye Kilburn, Gunnar Heuser, and William Spindell as "novel" and "unsupported by research extraneous to the litigation." Although a study by Kilburn had been published in a peer-reviewed journal, the court distinguished "editorial" peer review from "true peer review" and concluded that Kilburn's study suffered from "very serious flaws." [No. CV-S-92-0887-ECR, D. Nev. April 12, 1996]

Appendix G

Disciplinary Proceedings against
Hal A. Huggins, D.D.S.

In November and December 1995, the Colorado State Board of Dental Examiners held twelve days of hearings related to complaints brought against Dr. Huggins. On February 29, 1996, Administrative Law Judge Nancy Connick recommended that Huggins's license should be revoked. Huggins did not appeal, and his license was subsequently revoked.

The judge's 71-page report contained 235 findings of fact, some of which are excerpted below, together with the full text of the judge's conclusions. Copies of the full document are available for $12 from Quackwatch, P.O. Box 1747, Allentown, PA 18105.

Findings of Fact

4. For the past 22 years, Respondent [Huggins] has limited his practice of dentistry to the diagnosis and treatment of patients he believes are mercury toxic due to the placement in their mouths of dental amalgam fillings that contain mercury.

6. Respondent originally used amalgams in his dental practice. As early as 1973 Respondent became aware of anecdotal cases of medical improvements reported on removal of amalgams. Respondent states that he then began to observe similar phenomena in his own practice. It was at this time that Respondent adopted as his life's prime objective "exposure of mercury's destructive potential."

183

8. Respondent is the only dentist in the United States who trains other dentists how to treat patients with alleged mercury toxicity due to dental amalgams.

11. Over time the Huggins Center has had a staff of approximately 50 employees, including approximately three dentists; dental assistants; nurses (including a psychiatric nurse who assists patients who experience emotional upsets when their amalgams are removed); nutritional counselors; massage and movement therapists; a video producer; accountants; other business employees; and, for a while, a physician.

13. The Huggins Center accepts for treatment patients with just about any symptoms and . . . encourages prospective patients suffering from almost any illness to seek treatment from the Center and offers them assurances that their health will improve.

16. Many of the patients who seek treatment at the Huggins Center are very ill and are desperately seeking help.

17. The Huggins Center accepts the patient's medical diagnosis (e.g., multiple sclerosis), makes a diagnosis of mercury toxicity, and then treats the purported mercury toxicity and medical disease.

22. On several occasions, Respondent has told patients that he had MS and was cured, even though in fact Respondent has never suffered from this disease.

23. Respondent has designed two separate "detoxification programs," offered at the Huggins Center. The first is a comprehensive in-office program for those with serious problems. This program generally lasts two weeks, although it takes three weeks for ALS and leukemia patients. The Huggins Center has approximately 250 patients a year in this in-office program. The cost of this program is about $6,000 plus charges for the actual dentistry. The second is an "assist" program to patients outside Colorado, those with more moderate problems, and those interested in prevention. The assist program costs approximately $380 plus charges for serum compatibility testing and dental work.

38. Respondent admits that he cannot prove the link between mercury from dental amalgam and disease but believes that he is entitled to rely on his clinical experience which suggests such a link.

39. When asked to state the scientific basis for his theories on mercury toxicity from amalgams, root canal extractions, and cavitations, Respondent was very vague. While able to identify a handful of studies on which he relied, he generally referred to thousands of publications in

his library which supported his position, although he had not supplied them to the Board in response to requests and could not identify them. He also sought to portray questions seeking to identify these studies as unreasonable by, for example, indicating that his goal is to treat patients and not to "rattle off" citations in the literature. In addition, he indicated his philosophy that the absence of proof is not the proof of absence.

40. It is highly probable that had additional studies lent credence to Respondent's practices, he would have supplied them or at least been able to identify them in substantially greater detail, particularly in light of the fact that he knew the scientific bases of his practices were being questioned and his dental license was at stake.

72. Respondent testified that there are thousands of articles which establish that amalgam causes multiple sclerosis but was unable to give citations "off the top of his head."

87c. Respondent consistently represents that the Huggins Center has an 85 percent success rate, measured by an improvement in patient symptoms and chemistries. Respondent believes that his treatments are effective and that it is only the patient's unwillingness to continue adequate nutritional and other follow-up or the patient's falling into the unlucky 15 percent which prevents success. Because there is no scientific basis for the diagnosis or treatment performed at the Huggins Center, this statement is misleading, deceptive, and false.

89. As its standard protocol, the Huggins Center extracts all teeth which . . . have had root canals performed on them, even when they are asymptomatic.

110. As part of his diagnosis of mercury toxicity, Respondent uses a mercury toxicity questionnaire involving approximately 500 very general questions which are not connected to mercury toxicity and which have no diagnostic value. For example, the questionnaire inquires whether a patient has ever experienced emotional irritability, but this is not a sign or symptom of mercury toxicity.

169a. Respondent represents that both massage and sauna help remove toxins from the body. Respondent represents that sweating from a sauna aids a normal excretory mechanism of the body and removes mercury. . . . Respondent admits that there is no scientific evidence supporting his contentions in relation to sauna but relies on his experience. There is no scientific evidence that mercury is eliminated from the body through perspiration.

Conclusions of Law

1. The Board has jurisdiction over Respondent, his license, and the subject matter of this proceeding.

2. In relation to Count I, since July 1, 1986, in his book, publications, and videotapes, Respondent has engaged in advertising which is misleading, deceptive, and false in violation of Section 12-35-118(1)(k), C.R.S. (effective July 1,1986). . . .

3. In relation to Count II and specifically patients D.A., G.B., M.B., A.G., H.G., H.S., G.S., and Dr. T.F., Respondent has engaged in acts or omissions which fail to meet generally accepted standards of dental practice or which constitute grossly negligent dental practice, in violation of Section 12-35-118(1)(a), C.R.S. (1995). . . .

4. In relation to Count III, since July 1, 1986, Respondent has practiced dentistry as a partner, agent, or employee of or in joint venture with any person who does not hold a license to practice dentistry in Colorado or has practiced dentistry as an employee of or in joint venture with a partnership, association, or corporation other than as provided in Section 12-35-112, C.R.S., a violation of Section 12-35-118(1)(9), C.R.S. (effective July 1, 1986).

5. In relation to Count IV and specifically patients D.A., G.B., M.B., A.G., H.G., H.S., G.S., and Dr. T.F., Respondent has abandoned his patients by failing to provide reasonably necessary referrals to licensed physicians for consultation or treatment in violation of generally accepted standards of dental practice and in violation of Section 12-35-118(1)(v), C.R.S. (1995). . . .

6. In relation to Count V and specifically patients D.A., G.B., A.G., H.G., H.S., G.S. and Dr. T.F., Respondent has engaged in willful and repeated ordering and performance, without clinical justification, of demonstrably unnecessary laboratory tests or studies; the administration, without clinical justification, of treatment which is demonstrably unnecessary; the failure to perform referrals when failure to do so is not consistent with the standard of care for dentistry; and the ordering or performing without clinical justification of services and treatment which is contrary to recognized standards of the practice of dentistry as interpreted by the Board, in violation of Section 12-35-118(1)(x), C.R.S. (effective July 1, 1989). In relation to M.B., the only treatment rendered after the effective date of Section 12-35118(1)(x) was the prescription of supplements, which constitutes a violation of this section. . . .

7. In relation to Count VI, the above violations of the Dental Practice Law also constitute violations of Section 12-35-118(1)(h), C.R.S. (effective July 1, 1986).

Initial Decision

Once violations of Section 12-35-118(1), C.R.S., have been established, the Administrative Law Judge must determine what disciplinary sanction, if any, is appropriate. Such sanctions may be suspension of a license for a period of not more than one year; revocation of a license; or reprimand, censure, or probation. Section 12-35-118(1), C.R.S. In this matter, the Board's counsel seeks revocation of the Respondent's license. Respondent asserts that no discipline is appropriate.

In his practice of dentistry at the Huggins Center over the years, Respondent has engaged in a pattern and practice of violating the Dental Practice Act. He first engages in deceptive advertising to entice patients to seek dental treatment for their serious medical problems when in fact there is no known link between their teeth and general health or between the treatment offered and any improvement in their health.

The efficacy of this deceptive yet seductive advertising is shown by the thousands of telephone calls coming into the Huggins Center every month.

Respondent instills fear in the public that the mercury in their amalgams is poisoning their bodies. His emotionally charged publications, laced with scientific references and terminology, are designed to convince the public not only that amalgams are the undiscovered cause of everything from MS to Alzheimer's disease, but that there is a simple cure which offers them an amazing and tantalizing 85 percent success rate. The Huggins Center holds the key to their improved health.

Respondent offers hope not just to a few. His espoused treatment offers to remedy a host of conditions, including tremors, seizures, MS, ALS, Alzheimer's disease, emotional disturbances, depression, anxiety, unprovoked suicidal thoughts, lupus, scleroderma, rheumatoid arthritis, unexplained heart pains, high and low blood pressure, tachycardia, irregular heartbeat, osteoarthritis, chronic fatigue, "brainfog," digestive problems, and Crohn's disease. The sheer breadth and number of these diseases is staggering. They include a number of life-threatening and debilitating conditions for which medical science offers only symptomatic treatment. When faced with these serious diseases, it is no wonder that patients are willing to grasp at any hope of improvement and turn to Respondent for the miraculous improvements he promises. The debilitating nature of the diseases for which Respondent offers treatment and the desperate straits of a number of his patients, combined with the lack of any scientific basis for the treatments he offers, make Respondent's conduct particularly egregious. Respondent has taken advantage of the hope of his patients for an easy fix to their medical problems and has used this to develop a lucrative business for himself.

The diagnostic techniques and treatments offered by Respondent at the Huggins Center are scientifically unsupported, without clinical justification, and outside the practice of dentistry. The standard protocols which Respondent has developed thus provide care which does not meet generally accepted standards of dental practice and, in many cases, is grossly negligent. Instead of referring patients to physicians who could actually treat their underlying medical diseases and who could make a diagnosis of the mercury toxicity which Respondent suspects, Respondent simply ignores the limits of his qualifications and licensure and proceeds to treat these patients. He subjects patients to a wide array of tests and treatments which have no clinical justification.

In relation to the eight patients at issue here, Respondent used his standard protocols. While all these patients suffered financially due to Respondent's intervention, a number of them also suffered physically or emotionally. Respondent's encouraging D.A. to believe in her son's wish that she sell her wheelchair is so out of proportion to any benefit which could be anticipated that it is cruel. The Huggins Center treatment caused actual harm to A.G.'s mouth and gums, as well as her appearance, under circumstances when her prognosis was very poor. Far from affording her the hoped-for improvement of her liver cancer, the Huggins Center treatment actually diminished her well-being during the last months of her life. In relation to H.S., the Huggins Center diagnosis of her being very sick, coupled with the disclaimer of any liability if she proceeded without full treatment, caused her to transfer to the significantly more expensive in-office program and to experience emotional upset, which was aggravated when she was later told she had cancer.

Along the way, Respondent has clearly become convinced that his treatments are effective and that it is only the patients unwilling to continue adequate nutritional and other follow-up or those unlucky

15 percent who will not benefit from his treatment. He is perfectly capable of ignoring the large body of scientific evidence which suggests that his theories in every arena are not credible; citing scientific literature selectively; exaggerating findings or studies which appear to support his work; referring to the thousands of publications which support him yet being unable to produce those; and asserting that his clinical experience, as biased and unscientific as that may be, is itself the only support he needs. Respondent essentially says "trust me" to the dental profession and the public but provides no reasonable basis upon which he should be trusted.

Given his steadfast and longstanding commitment to his theories in the face of substantial reasoned evidence to the contrary, it is evident that nothing will stop Respondent from practicing the treatments he has developed short of revocation of his license to practice dentistry. Such disciplinary action is also justified by the multiple violations of the Dental Practice Act proven in this matter, especially those involving grossly negligent care.

Accordingly, it is the Initial Decision of the Administrative Law Judge that Respondent's license to practice dentistry in the State of Colorado is revoked.

Appendix H

Testimony of Gulf War Veteran Brian Martin*

Appreciation

Thank you, Mr. Chairman, and honorable committee members, for asking me to testify before you again today. I would also like to thank Congressman Upton for his continuous support and leadership, not only for the veterans of his district, but for all veterans across this great country.

Introduction

My name is Brian Martin. I am 33 years old. I am a husband, a father of two, and a Gulf War veteran. I am also a former member of the 37th Engineer Battalion, whose last mission of the 1991 war was to detonate and destroy an Iraqi ammunition depot called Kamasiyah. Tall Al Lahm to most of us, was where the huge ammunitions supply point was located in Iraq. There were 100 huge bunkers inside Kamasiyah and 43 metal

*Reproduced exactly as published in *The Status of Efforts to Identify Persian Gulf War Syndrome: Hearings before the Subcommittee on Human Resources and Intergovernmental Relations of the Committee on Government Reform and Oversight, House of Representatives, March 11, 28; June 25; and Sept. 19, 1996.* Washington, D.C.: U.S. Government Printing Office, 1997:323–325. This statement was presented on September 19th, when Martin was co-president (with his wife) of International Advocacy for Gulf War Syndrome.

pole-barn warehouses located just outside the depot's perimeter fence. We received the orders for this mission March 1st, 1991, during the cease-fire.

Kamasiyah

When our unit received the mission to move into Tall Al Lahm, our battalion commander separated the combat essentials and non-essentials for this mission. He sent the non-essential back to Rhafja, Saudi Arabia, while the rest of us (essentials) moved northeast to Kamasiyah. About 150 soldiers were used for this mission.

On March 3rd, 1991 we entered the bunker compound securing the area free of Iraqui civilians and rebels looking for ammunition to fight Saddam's republican guards. On March 4th, 1991, we re-entered the depot area, placing C–4 and Russian C–3 explosives in and around 33 bunkers, we set time charges for detonation, then moved SOUTH three miles to what we considered a "safe zone" as we waited for the anticipated explosions.

Detonation

From three miles away, we casually moved around taking pictures, recording video's and writing home. At no time whatsoever did we fear or have reason to fear chemical exposure. We were told by the 18th Airborne Corps that there were no chemicals in the area. We were told by the E.O.D. (Explosive Ordinance Disposal) team to simply "Blow it." That to our knowledge was the only so called "experts" in the area. No one in the 37th was chemical experts. For the record, our commanders knew nothing about chemicals in those bunkers. Seven minutes later, the destruction of Kamasiyah began.

During the Explosions

Getting excited as one could get, witnessing these awesome explosions was a remarkable sight. The explosions blew straight into the air and then would spread at the top. Many of us joked that this would be the closest thing to a nuclear mushroom cloud that we would see or ever hope to see. But our excitement quickly turned to fear when "cook offs" from the explosion began showering down on us. Several missiles landed underneath our trucks, spinning and taking off until blowing up. Men were running everywhere for cover. Hiding behind our vehicles for safety, we felt all hell had broken loose. With the dangers of being killed by the "cook offs" and the obvious giant clouds that were covering us, our battalion XO (executive officer) decided it was time to move us to a safer place to wait.

The 307th Engineer Battalion from the 82nd Airborne Division radioed to us, asking that we stop the detonation because of "cook offs" penetrating their area, making it extremely dangerous to complete their missions at Tallil Air Field. Tallil Airfield was over 12 miles away to the northwest, so our battalion XO decided we needed to move farther away than 12 miles. 20 miles later, he found an area that had no signs of "cook-offs" to the SOUTHWEST. Our battalion moved into convoy formation and proceeded to vacate the area.

For the next three days, it rained harder than any of us had seen in the 6 months we were there. Our commanders joked about us "putting something into the air to change the weather." For the next five days it was unsafe for us to return to Kamasiyah to finish destroying the remaining 67 bunkers. The skies were dark gray and cloudy for those five days.

Illnesses Since

Since just before those days at Kamasiyah, I have suffered from symptoms and ailments that have altered everything about me and my family's lives. It started in early 1991 with blood in my vomit and stools, blurred vision, shaking and trembling like I was on a caffeine high. My muscles were weakening, my chest pounded like my heart was going to explode through my chest. On Fort Bragg, during PT (physical training), I would vomit chem-lite looking fluids every time I ran, an ambulance would pick me up, putting IV's in both arms and rushing me to Womack Community Hospital. This happened EVERY morning after my return from the war. My symptoms were simply written off as a "stomach viral infection of an unknown origin." I was not allowed to advance in rank or transfer units due to my medical problems.

In December 1991, I put in for an "early out" from the military that I had loved so much. I did not receive an exit exam nor did I know that I was supposed to. I was told not to have children or give blood for 1 year. My medical conditions were ignored.

The Present

Today, as I have for the past five and a half years suffer from the symptoms that render me disabled. In a deranged way I guess I am lucky. I have some clearly defined diagnoses from the VA of MULTIPLE CHEMICAL SENSITIVITY, INFLAMMATORY BOWEL DISEASE w/scarring of THE COLON AND STOMACH due to chemical exposure, TEMPORAL LOBE BRAIN DAMAGE also w/scarring due to chemical exposure. I have REITER'S SYNDROME, CHRONIC FATIGUE SYNDROME and TINNITUS. I have a lower back condition which is quite painful, and abnormally high levels of pH Alkaline in my semen. I have abnormally high platelets around my blood cells and recently I began testing for LUPUS and Alzheimer's disease. From the first day I went into the VA in Battle Creek, Michigan, my records stated that I was exposed to something of an environmental contaminant during my service in the Gulf War. Recently, I underwent removal and biopsies of moles. I've had spots burned off my forehead with liquid nitrogen, and a spot in the middle of my back is presently under observation. Surgery is being scheduled to remove three lumps that are in my thigh, stomach and rib cage.

Even more recently, the VA has removed me from the permanent and total disability list, which I've been on since March 1996, forcing me to undergo all the Compensation and Pension (C&P) exams over again. From Louisville, Kentucky, to Washington, DC the VA computers claim that I am P&T (Permanent and Total). I have been approved for $30,000 life insurance from the VA, something that only a permanently disabled veterans receive. But one man Bob Marks who works for VA Adjudication Board in Michigan, claims I am not permanent or total. I was asked by the VA to apply for benefits for my family, something else a veteran cannot get unless he's permanent. When I argued this with Mr. Marks, he added a mental evaluation to my exams and said that "Chronic Fatigue

Syndrome is a mental disorder and not a physical one." The doctors that examined me in Battle Creek for these C&P exams all stated that this was a "waste of time and money for us all." For the first time in a long time I agreed with the VA doctors. With the help of Congressman Upton's office and hopefully this committee, Mr. Marks will be kept at bay.

For the last five and a half years, I suffer from excruciating painful headaches, memory loss and severe diarrhea. My family lives with my bad mood swings like walking on eggshells. I can no longer eat or drink many of the things that I used to. If I smell perfumes, vapors or chemicals that do not agree with my smelling senses, I violently vomit. I get lost when I drive sometimes and forget where I am at sometimes. I am an ex-paratrooper who needs a cane and a wheelchair to get around. My joints in my knees, hands, and knuckles swell, burn and hurt. My feet burn and swell if I spend anytime on them at all. My discharge summary from the VA (in 1993) states that I cannot sit or stand for prolonged periods of time. I am fatigued and feel worn out all the time, but yet I am an insomniac. For all of this except the chemical injuries and so much more, the VA has rated me in 1994 at 100% plus special monthly compensation, then in 1996 added the Permanent and Total, which is now being threatened.

My rating is 100% for Reiter's syndrome, 50% for chronic fatigue syndrome, 30% for colitis, 10% for tinnitus and 10% for lower back condition. Nothing for chemical injuries or illnesses. Zero's across the board for everything else. Since the admission of Kamasiyah, I thought the VA would've taken me a little more serious, instead, they're trying to take away my service-connected disability benefits. The only means of income my family has to pay our bills, clothe our bodies and feed ourselves. Instead of compassion, I received a police report, where the VAMC in Battle Creek, MI claims that they are going to press charges on me for cassette taping a doctor pushing my wife on VA property. Please help me figure that one out!

Conclusion

In conclusion, I would like to add that my wife and I have looked for the truth about our illnesses. We have always been honest and up front with the VA and the DoD. We have offered the videotape of Kamasiyah to anyone who wanted it. My chemical injuries do exist, they have since 1991. They've existed for the same five years and 110 days the Pentagon to the White House claimed that they knew nothing about Kamasiyah. They've existed for the same amount of time brave young veterans have died and scared young wives buried them. Their existing and we veterans learned to adapt to them, our pain has forced us to tap the resources of our spirits. My wife and measure our intelligence not by what we know, but by the way we view things. Everything we have endured for the past five and one half years has taught us the difference between a obvious downright cover up of corrupt disregard for human life, and the Veterans Affair's, simply put, gross incompetence. The right hand does not know what the left hand is doing and using DoD's ghost documents and ridiculous memorandums as their medical care guides is ludicrous. I've wondered how civilian doctors treat patients without the Pentagon sending them a memorandum explaining what couldn't have possibly happened to that patients. Medicine is indeed perplexing!

Observations

It amazes me to sit back and listen to all the different excuses the Pentagon has for messing up Kamasiyah. Are they frantic because we're exposed to a terrible chemical and are ill from it? or because they got caught denying it? The Pentagon recently said they didn't know American troops were in the area, but yet a general from the 18th Airborne Corps, can order a 900 man battalion to do a mission labeled as the largest man made explosion of the war, and there's no paperwork on it? Stephen Joseph testified to the P.A.C., that they uncovered their own cover up. I don't suppose the 1994 and '95 UN reports on Kamasiyah and my video tape had anything to do with it. If I had given the Pentagon that video tape in March when they pressured me for it, I believe their admission on June 21st would've never happened. But if they are the gallant ones, is it because enough of us have died and are sick enough to convince them their experiments and blatant cover ups have failed?

LTC. Jimmy Martin, who was with Stephen Joseph's Persian Gulf Investigation Team, claimed there are "thousands of documents in boxes, that they don't have the manpower to look through." Give them to me, we will look at them, it's important to all who suffer. Reading the memorandum stating that certain documents should not be put on the Gulflink*, why would they want to hide documents from the press or general public that describe certain important events? They have made their own bed of cover up and after the VA tucks them in, they must lay in it. These are the things that the DoD does to prove their intent to conceal proper information from the press, the veterans and you, the United States Congress.

I hope these hearings and this committee can help veterans mold a new reality for the Department of Defense and the Department of Veterans Affairs. A wake up call if you will. The support from the press, Congress and the American people is strong enough to convince these departments to listen to the veterans. If we are too ill or don't live long enough to enjoy the freedoms we have as Americans, what good was fighting for them?

---

*Authors' note: GulfLINK is the official World-Wide Web information service from the Office of the Special Assistant for Gulf War Illnesses in cooperation with the Defense Technical Information Center. Its purpose is to provide the public with recently declassified documents that may have potential relevance to the illnesses affecting Gulf War veterans. Its URL is http://www.gulflink.osd.mil/

Appendix I

Reputable Consultants

Scientific Experts

Robert S. Baratz, M.D., D.D.S., Ph.D.
159 Bellevue Street
Newton, MA 02158
(617) 332-3063

Ronald E. Gots, M.D., Ph.D.
International Center for Toxicology
    and Medicine
6001 N. Montrose Road, Suite 400
North Bethesda, MD 20852
(301) 230-2999

Thomas L. Kurt, M.D., M.P.H.
3645 Stratford Avenue
Dallas, TX 75205
(214) 528-3585

Herman Staudenmayer, Ph.D.
Behavioral Medicine & Biofeedback
    Clinic of Denver
5800 East Evans Avenue
Denver, CO 80222
(303) 758-8934

Abba I. Terr, M.D.
450 Sutter Street
San Francisco, CA 94108
(415) 433-7800

Legal Experts

William Custer, Esq.
Powell, Goldstein, Frazer & Murphy
161 Peachtree Street, 16th Floor
Atlanta, GA 30303
(404) 572-6600

Timothy E. Kapshandy, Esq.
Sidley & Austin
One First National Plaza
Chicago, IL 60603
(312) 853-7643

Bonnie Semiloff, Esq.
Spriggs and Hollingsworth
1350 I Street, N.W.
Washington, DC 20005
(202) 898-5823

Public Policy Consultant

Cindy Lynn Richard
Environmental Sensitivities
    Research Institute (ESRI)
5570 Sterrett Place, Suite 208B
Columbia, MD 21044
(410) 740-8922

Glossary

agoraphobia: Emotional disorder in which irrational fear of open or public places is so pervasive that the afflicted individual avoids or is reluctant to enter into a large number of situations. The term "toxic agoraphobia" has been suggested to characterize MCS patients who have become fearful about chemical exposure and have become socially withdrawn.

allergy: Abnormally high reactivity to specific antigens, brought about by immunologic mechanisms. Common allergic symptoms include rash, watery eyes, and wheezing. True allergies provoke a physically identifiable response.

amyotrophic lateral sclerosis (ALS): Progressive degenerative disease of the spinal cord that causes muscle weakness and atrophy and is usually fatal within two to four years; commonly called "Lou Gehrig's disease."

anaphylaxis: Sudden, life-threatening allergic reaction characterized by a sharp drop in blood pressure, difficulty breathing, and hives; also called anaphylactic shock.

antibody: Protein, produced by the body, that combines with a foreign material (antigen) to neutralize the foreign substance.

antigen: Substance that, when introduced into the body, stimulates production of an antibody.

attention deficit disorder: Disorder, primarily occurring during childhood, characterized by impulsiveness, hyperactivity, and short attention span.

atopic dermatitis: Skin problem is characterized by itching, scaling, and flaking; sometimes called eczema.

B cell: A type of white blood cell (lymphocyte) that matures in the bone marrow and produces antibodies.

blinding: Experimental condition where a test takes place without the benefit of background information that might prejudice the outcome or result.

"canaries": Term, sometimes used to characterize MCS patients, alluding to the practice of using canaries in coal mines to detect gas that is toxic but odorless. The death of a canary would indicate that a toxic level was present and the workers should leave.

candidiasis hypersensitivity: Fad diagnosis based on the notion that multiple common symptoms are the result of sensitivity to the common yeast *Candida albicans.*

cavitation: Term used to describe the craters of "cavitational osteopathosis," an alleged condition said to arise when root-canal treatments produce jawbone "cavitations" that cause disease elsewhere in the body. Cavitational osteopathosis should be regarded as a "fad diagnosis."

challenge test: Deliberate exposure to a substance to evaluate whether it produces an adverse reaction.

chemical sensitivity: Alternative term for multiple chemical sensitivity.

Crohn's disease: A serious chronic disease of unknown cause in which the intestinal wall becomes inflamed and ulcerated. The main symptoms are fever, diarrhea, cramps, and weight loss.

clinical ecology: Pseudoscience based on the belief that multiple symptoms are triggered by hypersensitivity to common foods and chemicals.

complement: A complex system of proteins found in normal blood serum that combines with antibodies to destroy potentially harmful bacteria and other foreign material.

corticosteroids: Any of the steroid hormones produced by the cortex of the adrenal gland; or their synthetic equivalents.

cytokine: Chemical messenger, produced by various types of cells, that helps regulate immune function and other processes.

defendant (in a court case): The party a legal action is brought against.

desensitization: Series of injections that make someone nonreactive or insensitive to an antigen. The amount used is tiny at first and is gradually increased. Also called immunotherapy.

double-blind test: Experiment in which neither the experimental subjects nor those responsible for the treatment or data collection know which subjects receive the treatment being tested and which receive something else (such as a placebo).

encephalopathy: General term for brain disease.

environmental medicine: Term used to describe scientific approaches to environmentally related health problems. These approaches differ from the main tenets of clinical ecologists, who have co-opted the term to make themselves sound more respectable.

epigastric area: Upper portion of the abdomen between the rib margins.

etiology: Cause or origin of a disease.

fad diagnosis: Dubious diagnosis popularized by unscientific practitioners.

homeopathy: Pseudoscience based on the notion that a substance that produces symptoms in a healthy person can, if given in extremely small amounts, cure ill people with similar symptoms. Homeopathic practitioners theorize that the smaller the dose, the more powerful the effect—which is the opposite of what pharmacologists have demonstrated in dose-response studies. Homeopathic products are prepared by repeated dilution. Some are so dilute that no molecules of the original substance remain.

hypersensitivity: Abnormally high sensitivity. Commonly used as a synonym for allergy.

hypersensitivity pneumonia: Inflammation in and around the tiny air sacs (alveoli) of the lung caused by an allergic reaction to inhaled organic dusts or other agents. Frequent or prolonged exposure to these substances is usually necessary to bring about the disease.

hyperventilation syndrome: Condition in which anxiety produces overbreathing accompanied by lightheadedness, numbness and tingling of the hands and feet, and various other bodily reactions.

hypochondriasis: Morbid preoccupation with having a specific illness, not verified by medical investigation, that persists despite physician reassurance.

idiopathic: Of unknown cause.

idiopathic environmental intolerances (IEI): Term suggested for replacing MCS; an acquired disorder with multiple recurrent symptoms associated with diverse environmental factors tolerated by the majority of people and not explained by any known medical or psychiatric/psychologic disorder.

IgE: Abbreviation for immunoglobulin E.

IgG: Abbreviation for immunoglobulin G.

immunoglobulin: A type of antibody.

intracutaneous: Into the skin

intradermal: Into the skin.

Legionnaires' disease: Relatively dangerous type of bacterial pneumonia most commonly spread through air-conditioning systems.

leukocytes: White blood cells.

limbic kindling: Dubious theory that a portion of the brain (related to cognition, emotions, behavior, glandular function, and sense of smell) can become sensitized and cause symptoms after repeated exposure to low levels of chemicals.

Lyme disease: Spirochetal disease usually transmitted by deer ticks. (Spirochetes are corkscrew-shaped bacteria.)

megavitamin therapy: Questionable treatment using high dosages of vitamins, usually ten times or more times the Recommended Dietary Allowances (RDA) set by the National Research Council.

mercury amalgam: Blend of mercury, silver, tin, copper, and zinc used for "silver" fillings.

nasal: Pertaining to the nose.

neutralization: Dubious treatment procedure in which various amounts of an offending substance are given until a dose is found that provokes no symptoms.

nosologic entity: A disease or diagnostic category.

objective sign (of illness): Indication of disease apparent to others besides the person affected.

organic brain function: Physical functioning of the brain.

organic compound: Carbon-containing substance related to or derived from a living organism.

organic disease or disorder: Condition in which there are anatomic or pathophysiologic changes in some bodily tissue or organ, in contrast to a functional disorder; particularly one of psychogenic origin.

panic disorder: A condition typified by sudden attacks of incapacitating anxiety. The symptoms can include rapid pulse; pounding heart; rapid, shallow breathing; and a sense of doom.

PET (positron emission tomography): Imaging procedure that combines the use of radioactive substances and computers to produce vivid color-coded pictures of areas inside the body.

phenols: A class of aromatic organic compounds.

phobia: Persistent irrational fear that impels the person to avoid the feared situation(s) or object(s).

placebo: Inert substance given for its psychologically soothing effect or for purposes of comparison in an experiment.

placebo effect: Favorable response that results from the act of treatment rather than the treatment itself.

plaintiff (in a court case): The party that institutes a suit in a court.

polymyalgia rheumatica: Condition that causes severe pain and stiffness in the muscles of the neck, shoulders, and hips.

porphyrias: Rare metabolic disorders, usually hereditary, characterized by the presence of large amounts of porphyrin in the blood and urine. Their most common symptoms are hypersensitivity to sunlight, abdominal pain, constipation and diarrhea, and neurologic disturbances.

provocation: Dubious clinical ecology procedure in which substances are administered by injection or sublingually to see whether the patient's usual symptoms occur.

psoriasis: A skin disease characterized by recurring reddish patches covered with silvery scales.

psychogenic: Caused by emotional mechanisms.

radioallergosorbent test (RAST): Blood test used to detect IgE antibodies to specific allergens, which may help to diagnose an allergic skin reaction, seasonal rhinitis, or allergic asthma.

radioimmunosorbent test (RIST): Blood test used to measure the total amount of IgE antibodies.

retrovirus: Type of virus that stores genetic information as RNA (rather than DNA) and releases an enzyme (reverse transcriptase) that enables it to invade the DNA of other cells and be reproduced when the infected cells divide.

rhinitis: Inflammation of the mucous membrane (lining) of the nose, often due to an allergy to pollen, dust or other airborne substance.

safe house: Dwelling said to be built and furnished with "nontoxic" materials.

scleroderma: Chronic disease characterized by degenerative changes and scarring in the skin, joints, and internal organs.

serial dilution-titration: Dubious test in which increasingly concentrated dilutions of antigen extracts are injected into the skin to determine the starting and therapeutic doses for allergy shots.

serum compatibility test: Bogus blood test developed by Hal A. Huggins, D.D.S., that allegedly determines which dental materials are compatible with the patient's immune system.

sick building syndrome: Term used to describe nonspecific symptoms, for which no single cause can be identified, that arise where a problem of indoor air quality is suspected.

sign (of an illness): Objective (visible and/or measurable) indication of a health problem.

somatization disorder: Condition in which the body responds to stress by producing multiple symptoms similar to those of disease.

SPECT (single photon emission computerized tomography): Specialized nuclear scanning procedure that produces very detailed cross-sectional images of the body. SPECT scans are very expensive and are used primarily for research.

spreading: Dubious clinical ecology concept that sensitization to one chemical can cause hypersensitivity to unrelated chemicals.

subcutaneous: Under the skin.

sublingual: Under the tongue.

summary judgment: Court ruling that decides a case before it can go to trial.

symptom: Subjective indication of a health problem. (What the patient feels.)

syndrome: The group of signs and symptoms that characterize a disease, psychological disorder, or other abnormal condition.

T cells: A type of white blood cell (lymphocyte) that arises in the bone marrow and matures in the thymus.

tachycardia: Rapid beating of the heart (over 100 times per minute).

teratogen: Drug, virus, or other agent that causes abnormal fetal development.

total body load: Dubious clinical ecology concept based on the idea that biologic, chemical, psychological, and physical "pollutants" can add to or multiply each other's effects and produce symptoms when the total exceeds what a person can tolerate. Also called "total load."

urticaria (hives): Allergic reaction of the skin characterized by itchy, raised white lumps surrounded by an area of red inflammation.

volatile substance: Substance that evaporates readily at normal temperatures and pressures.

wheal: Small area of swelling on the skin, accompanied by itching, which can be produced by an insect bite, injection of an allergenic substance into the skin, another other type of allergic reaction, or certain skin diseases.

workers' compensation: Payment that must be made to an employee who is injured while working or becomes disabled in connection with work.

Index